MW00736596

NAKED

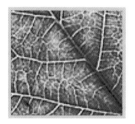

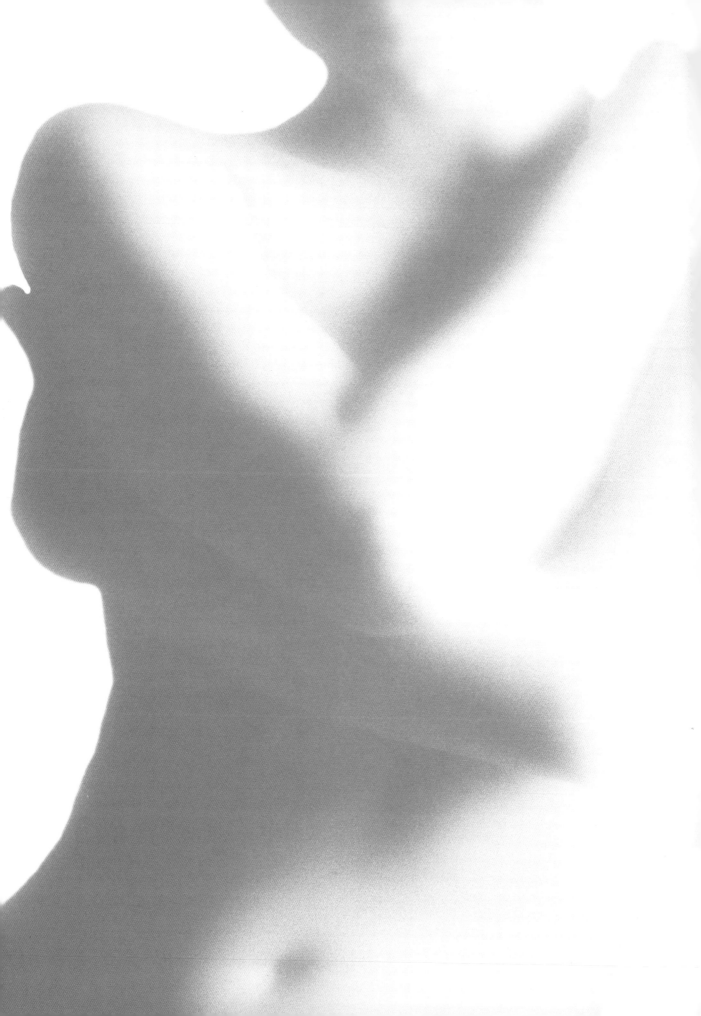

NAKED

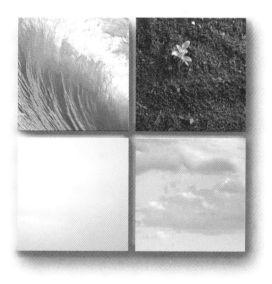

how to feel naturally healthy

linda gray

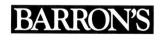

Contents

First edition for the United States, its dependencies, and
Canada published in 2002 by Barron's Educational Series, Inc.

Conceived and created by
Axis Publishing Limited
8c Accommodation Road
London NW11 8ED
www.axispublishing.co.uk

© Copyright 2002 by Axis Publishing Limited

All rights reserved.
No part of this book may be reproduced in any form, by
photostat, microfilm, xerography, or any other means, or
incorporated into any information retrieval system,
electronic or mechanical, without the written permission of
the copyright owner.

Creative Director: Siân Keogh
Designers: Juliet Brown, Sean Keogh
Project Editors: Matthew Harvey, Michael Spilling
Production Manager: Sue Bayliss
Photographer: Mike Good

Printed and bound by Star Standard Ind (Pte) Ltd, Singapore
9 8 7 6 5 4 3 2 1

All inquiries should be addressed to:
Barron's Educational Series, Inc.
250 Wireless Boulevard
Hauppauge, New York 11788
http://www.barronseduc.com

ISBN 0–7641–5515–6
Library of Congress Catalog Card Number 2002101226

introduction

In today's world, it can be easy to get lost in a sea of complications. It seems we have to go to

great effort to get back to what is natural, what is pure, and what is simple. *Naked* addresses

this ever-growing need, guiding you through different aspects of your life and exploring how

you can enjoy the goodness of simplicity. The book is divided into four sections, based on the

four classical elements, Water, Earth, Fire, and Air, which the Ancient Greeks viewed as the

fundamental building blocks of all matter and energy. In *Naked*, the four elements represent

four natural approaches to personal well-being. Water looks at how we can use this essential

substance to cleanse our lives, washing away mental and physical toxins. It helps you to explore

all the ways that water can enhance living, both in terms of cleansing, and restoring health and

well-being. Earth invites you to enjoy all the goodness and energy of the earth. This includes

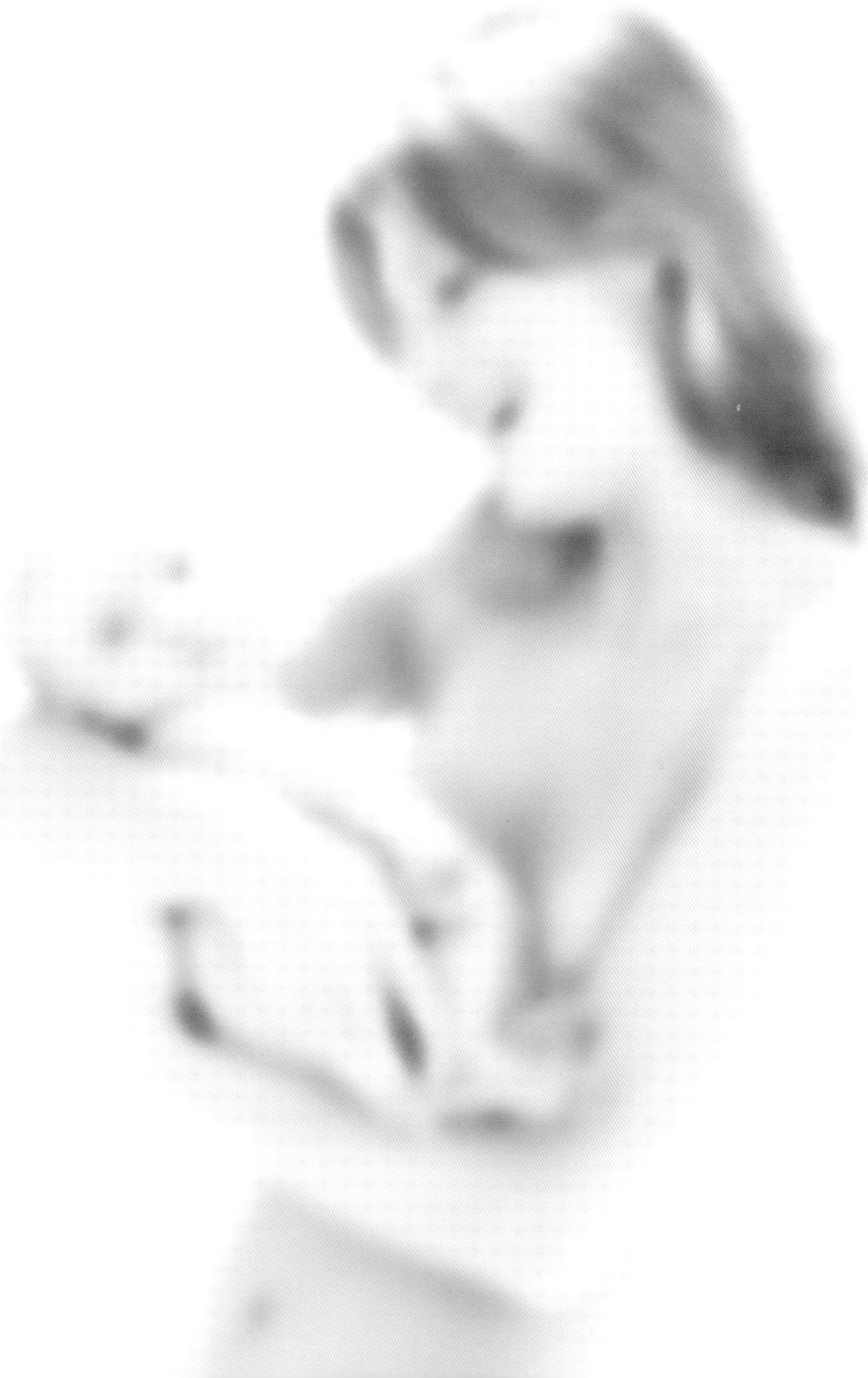

introduction

the substance of the earth itself as a cleansing agent and as a source of minerals. The chapter also looks at the foods that spring from the earth, and the many ways that we can enjoy the beneficial energy contained within them. Fire is about creativity and energy. It helps you to unleash your creativity and get your mind into a fertile, productive space. The chapter also explores how we can sustain positive energy within us to meet all the challenges and opportunities that life throws our way. Air deals with your connection to the spiritual aspects of yourself and looks at how you can achieve harmony and balance in your life. It explores the lessons to be learned in the simple act of breathing, and presents various methods of meditation. The chapter also discusses relationships and the ways that you can achieve balance within them. This chapter completes the mind, body, and spirit approach of the book.

So dip in or read the book from cover to cover. Each page will contain something to inspire you. As the pace of life gets ever faster, it is more important than ever for us to remember the important things in life, to keep things simple, and to be naked once again.

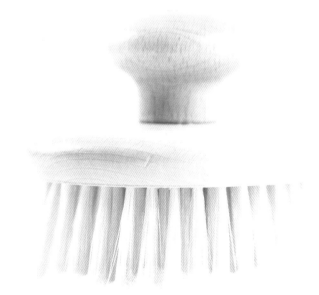

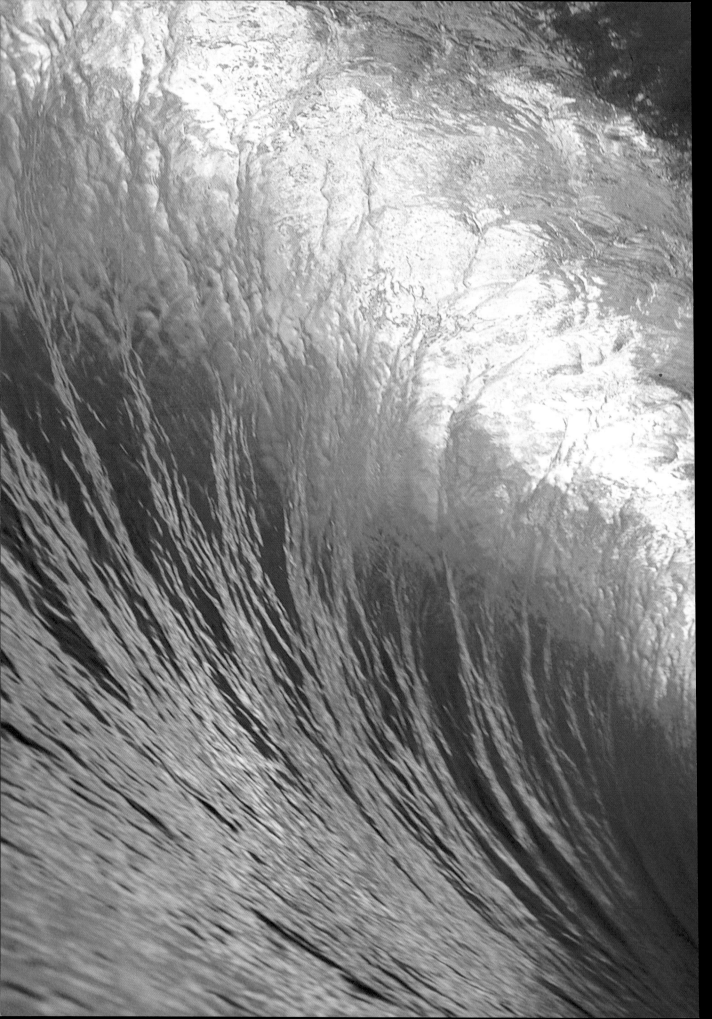

water

Life begins in water. Before birth, the waters of the womb modify our first sensations until we emerge into a world where water makes up two-thirds of the planet—and of our bodies. We recognize its fundamental importance by giving it a central place in many religious rituals. And yet this life-giving liquid is available simply by turning on a tap.

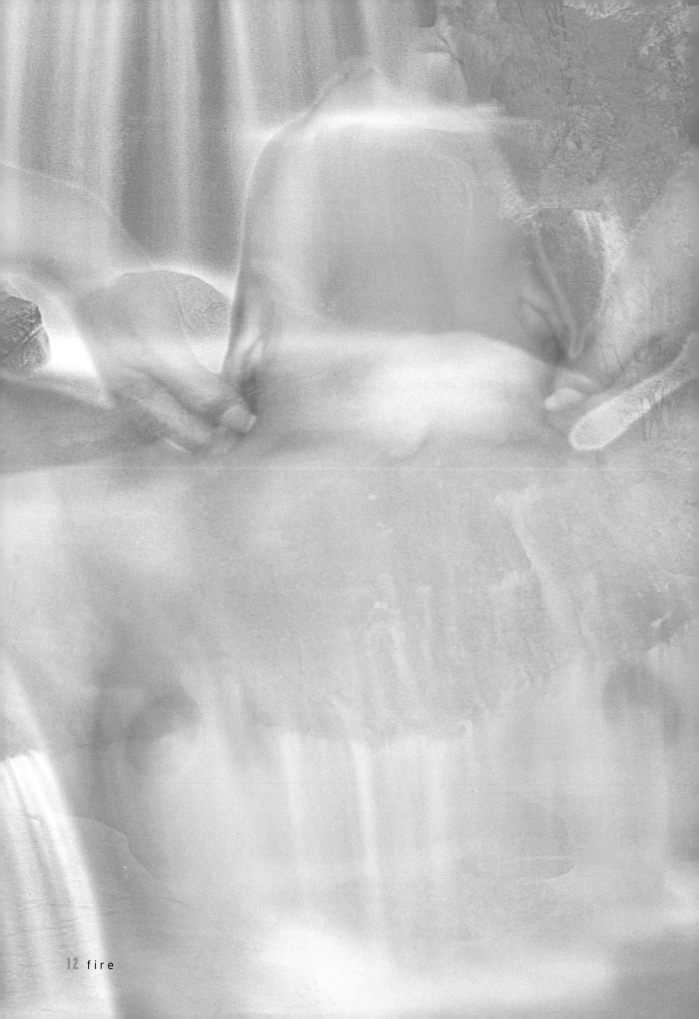

bathing

Rediscover the ritual of bathing. Floating naked in warm water is a shortcut to calm, returning you to the weightless, careless time before birth, stripping away grime from the body and stress from the mind in a process that cleanses both body and soul. And yet it can be difficult to focus and value the experience of bathing. Learn how to turn a hurried shower before leaving for work or a quick bath before going out in the evening into a moment of renewal.

water

sea of tranquillity

Think how the ocean can become a playground, a physical challenge, and a source of inspiration and you will

see how water can touch every part of your being, soothing skin and shaping muscles, refreshing

the spirit and relaxing the mind. Call on the inspirational and calming properties of the sea

every day by focusing on your senses while you bathe. The simple act of switching

off in the tub or shower, allowing your mind to think of nothing but being in

the moment, is a valid form of meditation.

surrender to the breath

As you enter the meditative state, concentrate on your breathing for a

few moments. Do not try to impose your will: Just allow the breath to

enter and leave your body like the waves washing onto the shore and

subsiding again.

leave the world behind

As you discard each layer of clothing, close your eyes and breathe deeply, clearing your mind of everyday stress and negative thoughts. Listen to the water as it runs into the bath and stir it with your fingers. Add a few drops of essential oil and breathe in its intense fragrance. Sink into the water and concentrate on your sensations—the way the languorous warmth of the water contrasts with the cooler walls of the bath, the scent and silkiness of the oils, the sounds of your breathing, and the sight of your arm, belly, or knee emerging from the water. Losing yourself in the moment like this is the essence of "flow," one of the principles of Buddhist vipassana meditation, and a great way to free your mind from invasive or troubling thoughts. Have a warm bathrobe waiting for you as you leave the bath. Avoid hurrying—take a few moments to re-engage with the physical world. This everyday ritual will leave you cleansed, refreshed, renewed, and ready for the world again.

water

the ultimate immersion

Buoyed up by a solution of salts and minerals so dense that you float effortlessly, and maintained at body-temperature so that you feel at one with the elements, you lie peacefully in the dark, cut off from all sound, until you reach a state of deep relaxation, even euphoria. Flotation therapy involves surrendering yourself to the water to the exclusion of all other sensory stimuli, and it is as close as you will get to being back in the womb.

when time stops

Allow yourself time for a few peaceful minutes first—you need a still, quiet atmosphere to achieve a receptive state of mind before lowering yourself into the water. Weightless and freed from even the tiniest distraction, you feel as if time is standing still, and as your heart rate and blood pressure drop, you experience a deep sense of calm. Aching muscles and joints experience a blissful release from tension and weight bearing.

trust the water

Some may feel a degree of bravery is required to undergo such an immersion, but there is nothing to fear. You are floating in less than a foot of water and it is always possible to switch on the light and leave the tank at any time. (Anyone susceptible to panic attacks or skin problems should take professional advice before trying flotation.)

If you do not feel ready to surrender all contact with the outside world, consider listening to a relaxation tape or combining flotation with hypnotherapy to make it easier to achieve that nirvana of calm.

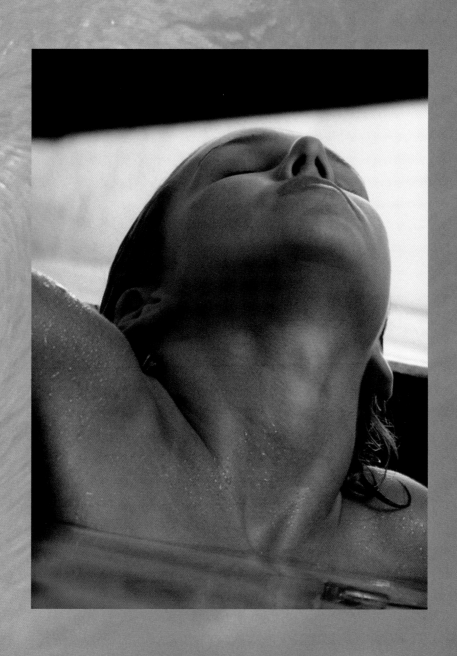

water

catch the tide

Water is ever changing and while it can mimic the peace of life before birth, it can also be a force that provides power to cities or forms the currents that shape continents. In its turn, water is controlled by the landscape that channels and filters it, and by the gravitational force of the moon.

creatures of the moon

The moon dictates the time of the tides and may also have an impact on our bodies. There is evidence that the structure of water is actually altered by the passing of the moon overhead. Little wonder then that we, who are two-thirds water, should be affected by its cycles.

Mere moonshine? Not at all. A paper published in the scientific journal *Nature* showed that growth in trees and even pot plants responds to tidal rhythms, and the maximum effect occurs at the full and the new moons. This raises the question of how the moon affects human health. It has long been thought to have a psychological link. The word "lunatic" is derived from the moon and there is some evidence that violence in jails and psychiatric hospitals increases at the time of the full moon. There could also be a physiological connection—at 28 days, the average female menstrual cycle is the same length as a lunar month.

a time to reap, a time to sow

The moon is an important element of folk medicine, where herbs are picked and planted and animals tended according to the phases of the moon. The new moon is seen as ideal for fasting and cleansing the system in preparation for the waxing (increasing) moon, which is thought to be the best time to rest and absorb energy, including food. In contrast, the waning moon encourages action and is considered the best time for surgery.

observing your rhythms

Keeping a moon diary may reveal subtle effects on your health. Write down your moods and feelings for 28 days, starting at the new moon, and analyze them to see if your appetite and energy reflect the waxing and waning moon.

water

ease body and mind

To unwind and combat stress, soak in a scented bath no warmer than skin temperature (93-94°F) for 15 to 20 minutes. Well-chosen herbs or essential oils will soothe your spirit and your body.

a soothing bath

Take a handful of herbs dried at home or from a herbalist, tie them in a muslin bag and put it into the bath or tie it to the tap so that the hot water flows through—chamomile, lavender, and passionflower are all soothing varieties. So is the ancient medicinal herb valerian, but its pungent scent means it is best mixed with sweeter-smelling herbs before adding it to your bath. Alternatively, use up to six drops of pure essential oils (four if you have sensitive skin), which affect the limbic area of the brain, controlling mood and emotions.

an uplifting bath

For a euphoric bath, aromatherapy guru Robert Tisserand recommends two drops of relaxing clary plus two of heady ylang-ylang. You can substitute two drops of healing lavender oil for more of the costly ylang-ylang if you prefer, plus one drop of uplifting orange oil to freshen the whole mixture.

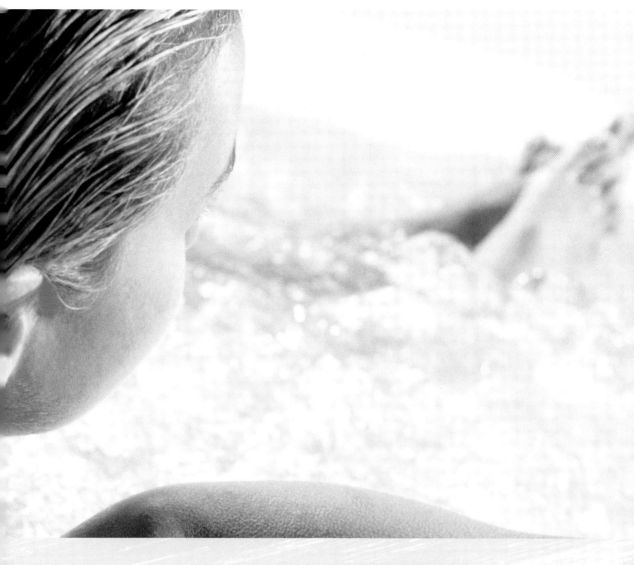

fill the senses

To intensify the effect of your scented bath, bathe by candlelight

and listen to music specially recorded for relaxation, which will

disengage rather than stimulate your mind.

water

and so to bed

From childhood, we associate bath time with bedtime—the mingled sensations of damp hair, the clean scent of soap and warm fresh towels, the cosseted, sleepy feeling as tired limbs sink into bed. But it is not just a learned habit—bathing really does help us begin the slide toward unconsciousness.

set the temperature

Your bath should be a bridge between the stimulations of the workaday world and the quiet of sleep, so extremes are out, such as water that is too hot or too cold. Warm water—but no warmer than 102-105°F (102°F if you're pregnant, elderly or suffer from high blood pressure or circulation problems)—induces relaxation and sleep, dilating the blood vessels and slowing the activity of the heart and lungs. Before getting into the bath, make sure everything is ready for the transition to bed. Make sure bathroom and bedroom are equally warm, and warm your towel, nightwear, and bed so that you move from one medium to the next without stimulating yourself.

sleeping potion

Blend two drops each of chamomile and sandalwood (an oil that is ideal for promoting sleep) and add them to the water. This bath is so soporific that it is wise to set your alarm or, better, get someone to rouse you gently after 15 minutes—after all, the aim is to fall asleep in bed, not in the bath.

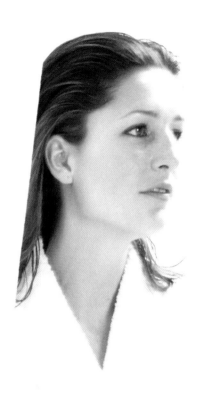

more sleeping potions

1 As well as chamomile and sandalwood, you

can add clary, sage or lavender to your bath

to help you sleep.

2 You can also try putting a few drops of

lavender oil on a handkerchief and keeping it

under your pillow as you sleep.

3 A traditional sleep aid is to soak the feet in

warm water. This draws blood away from the

head, so it can actually aid relaxation.

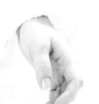

water

free from pain

Lying in warm water (a maximum of 105°F) encourages the brain to produce

endorphins, the body's own pain-relieving chemicals. It is a particularly

effective way to soothe the pain caused by such conditions as chronic

backache, tension headache, and period pain. Water also soothes pain by

activating the receptors in the skin and spinal cord. Do not underestimate the

power of water for pain relief—many women giving birth have found it so

effective that they needed no other analgesics. "Aromatic baths are useful in

the treatment of female disorders," said Hippocrates, the famous

fourth-century B.C. Greek doctor. For period pains, try adding essential oils of

clary and marjoram to a bath. For general aches and pains, make a lavender

rub for your temples and the nape of the neck by blending five drops of

lavender essential oil with a tablespoon of sweet almond oil; use this soothing mixture while soaking in a bath

to which you have also added two drops of chamomile, two of lavender, and one of orange essential oils.

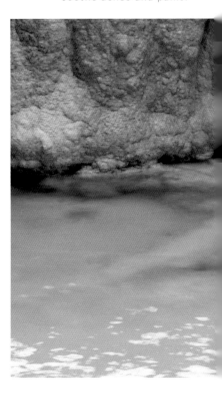

Water has a natural ability to soothe aches and pains.

unlock the power of water

To unlock tight muscles, sink into a whirlpool spa with adjustable jets to provide a soothing massage, or stand

beneath a pulsating shower for a similar effect. Although soft on contact, water can be imbued with enough power

to make it an effective massage tool—it is also a very pure way of applying force to the body. Hydrotherapy is

natural pain killers

all essential oils should be blended with a neutral carrier oil (about six drops of oil to four teaspoons of neutral oil before being applied to the skin.

headaches

lavender oil (massage), peppermint (steam inhalation), chamomile, ylang-ylang (bath)

backache

lavender, ginger, juniper, marjoram, rosemary (bath), black pepper (massage)

stomachache

angelica, melissa, peppermint, ginger, cardamom, basil, marjoram (massage)

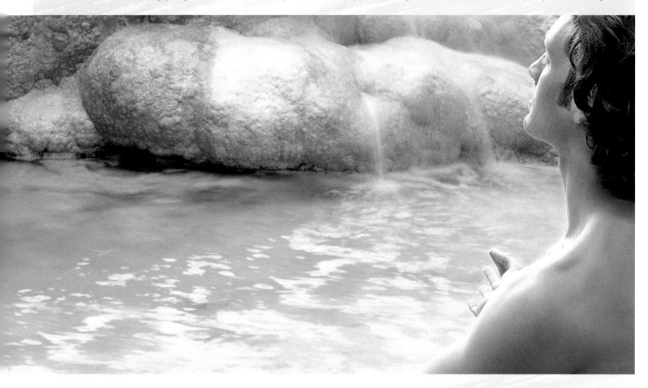

frequently recommended for severe chronic pain: Exercises in water kept at around 100°F rely on its buoyancy to cushion the joints and maximize the effect of physiotherapy. At home, gentle rinses can mimic the effect, using a pitcher, sprinkler, or hose to pour tepid water on the affected part of the body. As with any form of massage, work toward the heart from the extremities, moving the stream of water along one side of the arm, shin, face, or back and then the other.

heat and cold

Do not overlook the usefulness of a simple hot or cold compress in relieving pain. Ice packs for inflammation, bruising, and sprains and towels wrung out in hot water for aching joints and tension, are all effective traditional remedies.

water

winter wonder

When the days are short and the skies gray, we can feel sapped of energy and easily fall prey to opportunistic infections. Colds and flu can leave us feeling dehydrated, congested, and run-down. Water might seem an unlikely ally, but it can help to fight infection. Next time you feel the sore throat and stuffy nose that are the warning signs of a cold, add three drops of lavender oil and two of tea tree oil to your bath to help stop it from developing.

fighting the invader

Once you actually get a cold or flu, all you can do is to relieve the symptoms, which might include a mild fever and congested nasal passages. Sponging with cool (never cold) water is the recommended way to bring down a high temperature and many medical practitioners advise steam inhalations for blocked sinuses. Fill a bowl with freshly boiled water and lean over it, covering your head with a towel to contain the steam while you inhale. This traditional advice is backed by evidence from the British Cochrane Review of treatments, which found that in three trials, heated, humidified air eased the symptoms of the common cold.

Adding oils like lavender, tea tree, and eucalyptus, all of which have anti-infective properties, may do even more to shift congestion. Use two drops of each plus two of lemon.

A steam room invigorates and cleanses the body, while allowing moisture to be drawn in through the nose and lungs.

water

a shock to the system

A system of alternate warm and cool baths has been used for centuries to boost immunity. The theory is that while warm water opens up the blood vessels and helps eliminate waste, thereby improving immunity, cool water directs blood away from the skin and boosts the supply to the organs, a process called vasoconstriction, which helps prevent inflammation.

Manipulating body temperature with cold wraps is another way to increase resistance to infection, in healthy adults. Your body is wrapped in sheets wrung out in cold water, then immediately covered with dry towels and blankets. In most cases the body quickly regains its lost warmth and beneficial sweating begins, but extra warmth should be given in the form of a hot water bottle or a hot drink if normal temperature is not restored within 15 minutes.

kick start your body

A secondary effect of cold water is that it jerks the circulation into action, so in healthy people the initial chill is quickly followed by a rise in body temperature. Certainly, a splash of cold water after a warm bath is stimulating and helps boost supplies of energy. However, remember that complete

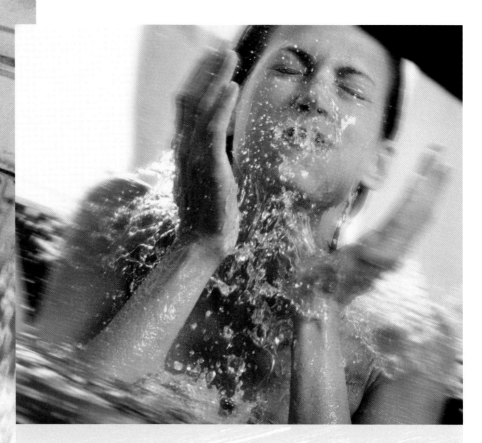

a gentler way

If you find the thought of a cold shower too brutal, try running cool water into the bath as you drain

away the warm, so that the temperature reduces gradually—do not stay in cold water too long,

though. Finish by spritzing your body with cool mineral water.

immersion in freezing cold water can be deadly, because it can stop the heart.

This cold shock response is less evident in those used to bathing in cold water

and the answer may be that becoming gradually accustomed to cold water

does indeed toughen you up...but a minute in a cold shower may be just as

effective (and safer) than a cold plunge into freezing water.

water

work out in water

We feel strange walking in water, our limbs unusually slow to respond—the overriding sensation is a combination of effort and lightness, like walking on the moon. Just as space travel cancels the effect of gravity, so the buoyancy of water makes us feel weightless. At the same time, though, muscles, circulation, and breathing must work harder than on land because water pressure is greater than that of air—so warming up is more important than ever when exercising in water.

work easier

The resistance of water is more than ten times that of air, so exercising in water can use 25 percent more calories than the same maneuvers carried out on dry land, which makes water the perfect element for increasing stamina. At the same time you can safely put more effort into your workout

Water increases the force required
for movement, while at the same
time reducing wear on supporting
joints such as the hips and knees.

because exercising in water reduces pressure on joints like hips and knees by 50 percent—up to 75 percent if you go more than waist deep into the water. Good exercises include walking (wear pool shoes if your feet slip), jumping imaginary rope, kickboxing, and resistance training. Excellent as it is for cardiovascular exercise like swimming and aqua aerobics, water is also the perfect medium for stress-relieving therapies such as t'ai chi and watsu (water shiatsu). Make sure that the water you are exercising in is clean and pure to minimize the risk of infection. The water should also be free of heavy doses of chlorine used for disinfection. This powerful chemical can irritate eyes and skin and cause drowsiness. Aqua aerobics has become a popular way to gain the benefit of exercise with reduced wear and tear on the body's frame. You don't even have to be able to swim well to take advantage of water fitness programs—they usually take place in the shallow end of the pool.

water

refreshing

Reach for water next time you need a lift. It is the perfect pick-me-up and a highly **effective** health and beauty treatment. As you drink, every cell and organ in the body drinks in moisture and nutrients. Water **lubricates** the joints, regulates body heat, and flushes impurities from the body. The result is increased energy, a sharper mind, smoother skin, and a brighter complexion. So have a drink by all means if you feel tired or stressed. Just make sure that it is clear, **pure** water.

water

thirst

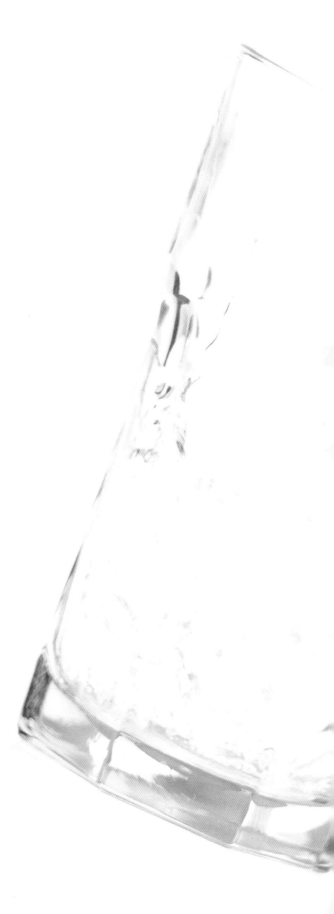

In the industrialized world, the endless task of providing water for us is assured. But we have not entirely lost our sense of its importance. Images of thirst and refreshment still hold their power for us. Wilting flowers, cracked dry earth, a parched tongue—all leave us with a feeling of unease. The shower of rain, the long cool drink of water, come as blessed relief and carry a promise that life can go on.

the thirsty spirit

Thirst is such a powerful idea—more so even than hunger, since we need water more than food—that we use it as a metaphor for intellectual and spiritual longing. We thirst for knowledge, for power, for life. We know that water can refresh the spirit as well as the body, which is why holy water and sacred springs play an important part in so many faiths.

meditate on water

Water promises us well-being. Our thought patterns take the form of waves, so perhaps it is not surprising that listening to the surge of the sea or watching a river flow can induce a state of contemplation and deep calm. In feng shui, the ancient Eastern art of living in harmony with universal energy, water is the great communicator. Feng shui practitioners recommend placing a dish of blue marbles on the highest surface in the room to draw on its energies, and placing shells, pebbles, and driftwood from the beach, and images of rivers and the sea around the home to bring the power of water into your life. The sound of moving water is also viewed as a highly energizing addition to a home or garden. The light, tinkling sound of water also helps to soothe the mind and promote deep relaxation.

water

health in a glass

getting enough

Quenching your thirst with cool water is one of life's pleasures. We depend on water to regulate temperature and carry away toxic wastes. Water also releases oxygen into our system. The body cannot store water for long—we lose about two cups a day just by breathing—and although a certain amount is obtained from food, a regular intake of four pints of pure water a day is required for good health.

But the pleasure you feel in quenching your thirst is a sign that your body is under stress. Thirst is not an adequate guide to when you need water. By the time you start to feel thirsty you may already be quite dehydrated, with flaking lips, a dry mouth and dark, strong-smelling urine—all signs that your body is crying out for water. If you wait until you are conscious of the need to drink, you could well consume less than half the amount recommended. So to get your daily four pints, aim for eight tall glasses of water during

benefits of water

Natural mineral water from bore holes and springs contains a wide variety of trace elements. While the chief benefit of drinking mineral water is the water itself (H_2O), these minerals can have health benefits. Mineral waters often contain CALCIUM: good for the bones and teeth; MAGNESIUM: helps to combat fatigue and stabilizes body temperature; POTASSIUM: important for muscles and movement; SODIUM: helps the body achieve a balanced water level; ZINC: used to build DNA, it increases healing of wounds (thus the salves containing zinc) and also regulates the insulin in the course of the day. A glass on rising and at bed-time, one at each meal plus one mid-morning, mid-afternoon, and mid-evening is not an impossible tar-get. And drinking water before each meal is a com-mon way to fill up if you have weight to shed. There is little need to exceed this unless you are exercising hard, if there is a heat wave, or you have a medical condition: People with a tendency to form kidney stones, for example, may be advised to drink more than twice as much.

the body; BICARBONATES and CHLORIDES: assist in regulating the acid levels in the stomach; FLUORIDE: helps preserve teeth from decay; and IRON: deficiency in iron can contribute to anemia. Read the label of mineral water bottles to find out exactly what each brand contains. The mineral content also affects the flavor of the water. The health benefits of the minerals in the water are never that great—so don't decide what to drink on the basis of what minerals a certain brand contains. Instead, use your taste buds to make your choice and buy what tastes best to you.

water

water of life

Drinking four pints of water a day is a simple prescription for health, but the first thing to emphasize is that it should be water that you drink, and still water at that—rather than tea, coffee, beer, wine, fruit juice, cola, nor even carbonated water. Here are some of the reasons why it is best to stick to plain water.

precious liquid

Water contains no caffeine, so every drop goes toward hydrating your body. Caffeine (found in tea, cola, and chocolate as well as coffee) is diuretic, so that welcome cup of tea or caffe latte is topping up your fluid levels by only half the amount you drink. Water contains no alcohol. Alcohol is even more diuretic than caffeine. For every unit of alcohol you drink, you lose the same amount of water (and gain a hangover).

nothing added

Water contains no sugar or sweeteners. Fruit juice may be a wonderful source of vitamin C, but like many soft drinks, it is packed full of sugar; a normal glass of fruit juice contains around 150 kcal. Sugar-free soft drinks usually contain synthetic sweeteners, which many health-conscious people try to avoid. Some sweeteners have been linked to cancer and are undergoing health reviews. The advice seems to be to avoid them until they are proved safe. Finally, carbonated drinks, have been shown to damage tooth enamel. Some studies, most recently in the United States, have also shown a link with bone fractures and it is thought that the acid carbonated drinks contain could affect the way the body metabolizes calcium. So make water your staple drink, and have the others just occasionally. Make plain tap water taste better by filtering it and keeping it in the refrigerator. Add a couple of slices of lemon or lime, plus ice if you prefer.

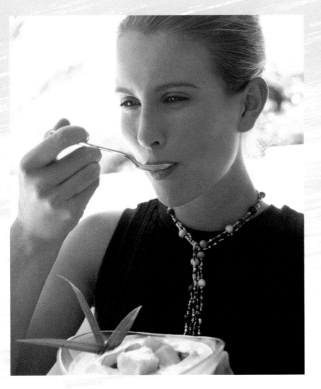

eat to drink

All foods contain water. Vegetables are a good source: Broccoli and carrots are 89 percent water, cucumber 96 percent. Most fruits contain around 75 percent water, and even bread (about 40 percent) and roast meats (around 50 percent) contribute.

water

pure and clean

water you can trust

Imagine if one day you turned on the taps to find that they had run dry. Where would be your nearest natural source of water, and how safe would it be? A consistent supply of clean water is one of the basic requirements of civilization, freeing us from the endless burden of finding and carrying water that takes up most of the day in many countries.

In most industrialized countries, the water supply has to meet stringent regulations. Microorganisms are one possible source of contamination, so chlorine may be added to prevent bacterial growth, though people with compromised immunity are advised to boil tap water before drinking it at all times. Chemicals, such as nitrates from agricultural fertilizers (which frequently seep into the water), are another concern, but the permissible levels in tap water are very low, and the supply is constantly monitored for contamination.

Depending on the source of the water, it may contain

useful levels of calcium, magnesium, potassium, and

iron. "Hard" water contains relatively high levels of

calcium and magnesium, both vital mineral nutrients.

These minerals are absorbed into the water while it is

in the ground, so water from different regions can

have quite different mineral contents.

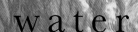

water

filtering

Why filter tap water? Some people are unhappy about chemicals such as fluoride and chlorine, which are added to the water supply for health reasons. Some substances may escape the water supplier's purification processes, including the heavy metals aluminum (used in processing tap water) and lead (used for water pipes in pre-war buildings—it can leach into the water with implications for memory and IQ, especially in children). Water in much of South America and Asia and parts of the United States can be affected by arsenic, found naturally in the earth's crust and also used in industrial processing, which is why the U.S. government recently announced measures to reduce arsenic levels by 80 percent. And the minerals in hard water can be a nuisance, encrusting heating elements in water heaters and coffee machines.

which filter?

A simple carbon jug filter will remove most contaminants, though not all. Keep the filtered water covered and store it in the refrigerator to keep it fresh. A water purifier fitted to the water supply works in the same way and means that filtered water is always on tap. Some claim to remove all particles, chlorine, and bacteria (including the lethal food poisoning microorganism *E.coli*), as well as over 90 percent of pesticides, heavy metals, and xeno-estrogens from industrial waste (which can affect our normal hormonal balance), plus 85 percent of nitrates. Look for independent checks before you buy. Not every filter will remove the bacterium cryptosporidium, which can escape the disinfecting process in reservoirs. For this you need a reverse-osmosis filter that meets the international standards set by the American National Standards Institute.

keep it clean

Bacterial growth in filters can confound all your efforts to safeguard

the purity of drinking water, so it is wise to follow instructions for

replacement carefully, and to do so with clean hands. And if you use

a filter that removes chlorine, you must keep the filtered water

refrigerated, or it will become a breeding ground for bacteria.

water

source of goodness

Deep underground, water emerges from beneath rock strata that formed in prehistoric times and wells to the surface, pure and clean, often as a bubbling spring. Such springs have long been a trusted source of drinking water. Some are famous for their health-giving properties, often attributed to high levels of certain minerals, and their water is bottled and distributed all over the world. As people have become more aware of the issues surrounding mass water supply and increasingly worried about contamination, many have turned to bottled water as an alternative. Sales of bottled water in the United States doubled between 1990 and 2000. However, comparing bottled with tap water is not straightforward. The purity and benefits of both kinds vary with the source and the processing. In the United States, about 25 percent of bottled waters are made from municipal water.

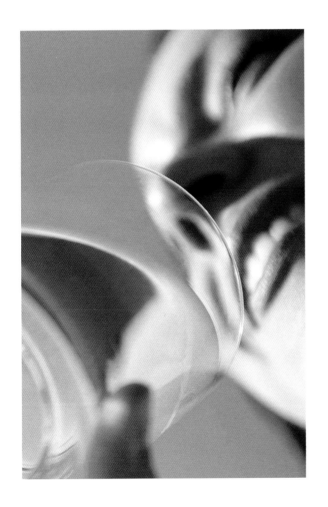

Most people find it reassuring that bottled water must, according to regulations, come from protected sources. Mineral waters must also contain minimum levels of certain minerals to qualify. Bottled water is regulated in the United States by the Food and Drug Administration.

Bottled waters usually offer superior taste. The softness of Badoit, the tang of Malvern, the stillness of Evian—to name just a few—make sipping a glass of water a delight.

water

coming clean

Soap yourself in the bath with a sponge and you remove waste that has been eliminated from within the body, as well as external dirt. The skin is the largest organ in the body and one of its most important functions is to rid the system of impurities brought to the surface by the network of pores and sweat glands. As you wash, the dirt is dissolved (by soap), detached (by friction), and finally rinsed away, leaving your skin glowing and refreshed.

Skin rescue

"Cleanse, tone, moisturize" is a mantra familiar to women throughout the developed world, and—despite a slew of specialized creams stuffed full of alpha-hydroxy acids, sun-protection factors and vitamins—the basis of a simple beauty routine followed by millions. Yet every part of it depends on one element: Water.

caring for your skin

Skin care works on the same principles. Facial washes, cleansing bars and cleansing creams contain detergents or oils to loosen the dirt—which is a mixture of skin debris, bacteria, sweat, and make-up—that is then removed by water, cotton wool, or cleansing cloths. Exfoliants—abrasive masks or facial scrubs

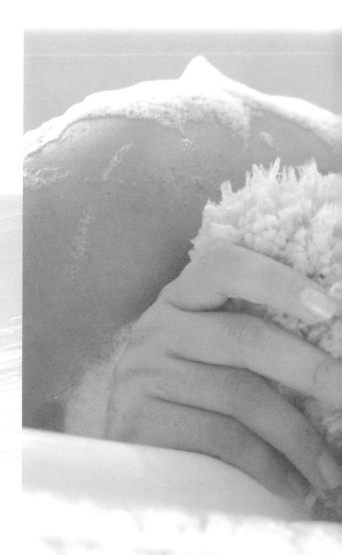

that help shift dead cells on the surface of the skin, revealing the fresh layer beneath—provide extra friction. Another way to intensify the cleansing process is to use water in the form of steam, which encourages the pores to open fully. (But avoid high temperatures, which can lead to damaged skin.)

Though cleanliness is essential, do not strip the skin of moisture. Soap is too harsh for many skins, which benefit from a gentler regime of pH-balanced facial washes and cream cleansers. The chief constituent of many of these is in fact "aqua"—water. So, why not try a homemade alternative? (See pages 48-49.)

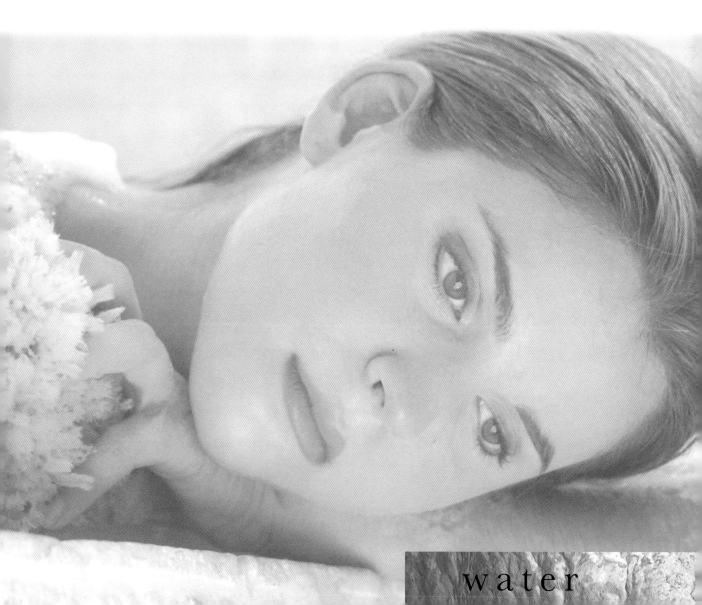

water

face and body cleansers

A good cleanser needs to be effective but gentle on your skin.

grape facial wash

Wine was used as a cleanser in eighteenth-century France, perhaps

because it contains fruit acids (AHAs), now known to have a natural

cleansing and peeling action. You can get the same benefits from

grapes (check a small patch on your skin for sensitivity). Wipe your

face with pure grape juice or use the cut side of large grapes.

Follow by rinsing your skin with plain water.

salt glow

This is a wonderfully invigorating natural exfoliant for the body that

leaves the skin radiant and silky smooth. Mix a cup of sea salt with

one cup of olive or almond oil—add a drop or two of lavender or

peppermint essential oil if you wish. Rub into the skin and then

shower away.

rolled oats facial scrub

Rolled oats are a traditional skin smoother. Mix two teaspoons of

fine rolled oats with one of baking soda and mix to a paste with a

little water. Rub gently into the skin, then rinse with cool water.

rolled oats bath powder

Mix together equal parts of rolled oats and powdered milk (which

contains cleansing lactic acid) in a blender. Place in a muslin bag

and add to the bath water for a relaxing soak.

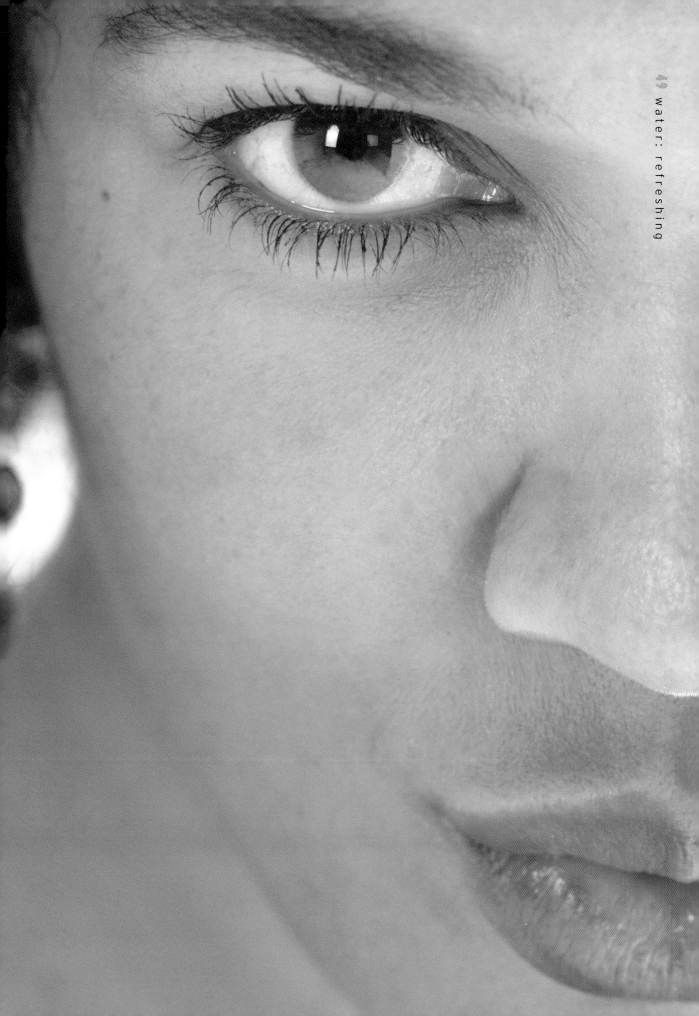

tonic for the skin

Rinsing and toning aim to close the pores after cleansing and to refine the skin. Always close the pores after cleansing to stop dirt getting in. Often, cool water is all that is necessary.

the right toner

Skin toning products are formulated to remove any traces of oil from the skin after cleansing. They are also astringent. This means they dry and shrink the surface tissues by reducing water content. If you have dry and sensitive skin, avoid any toner containing alcohol, which exacerbates dryness. If you have oily skin, a cotton ball wipe with toner will remove any residual oils after cleansing, but you may still find that astringents will sting, and too much toner can irritate the skin over time.

roses in your cheeks

Rosewater is an old-fashioned skin toner still available from some drugstores and specialized food stores. Traditionally, rosewater is what is left when essential oil of rose is distilled, but you can enjoy its healing, moisturizing, and antibacterial properties by making your own. Pour a pint of freshly boiled water over about three ounces of rose petals, leave to cool, and then strain. Add glycerin if your skin is dry or witch hazel if it is oily.

water

soft, supple skin

How do moisturizers moisturize? The answer is that on the whole they don't—they simply form a waterproof barrier that stops the skin from drying out. The richer the formulation, the thicker the barrier, which is why moisturizers for dry skins are much creamier than those recommended for oily skins.

Most skin creams have a moisturizing function but some specialized products, like serums to combat the signs of aging, skin firmers, and sun-protection creams, should be used in addition to moisturizer. If you opt for one of these, check whether it should be used over or underneath other creams for best results.

Night creams are simply extra-rich moisturizers. Primarily designed for mature skins, they were once heavier versions of what were called "day" creams. They still tend to be richer and often contain sophisticated ingredients designed to keep the effects of aging at bay.

natural hydration

Moisturizing face masks provide the most intensive treatment of all. For a natural face mask, mash an avocado (rich in vitamin E, the anti-aging vitamin) and apply thickly to your face and neck for 15 minutes. You can use avocado as a body butter, too. For extra hydration, rub it on and cover with cellophane wrap, then leave for an hour before showering. A little aloe vera juice or gel added to the avocado makes this even more soothing.

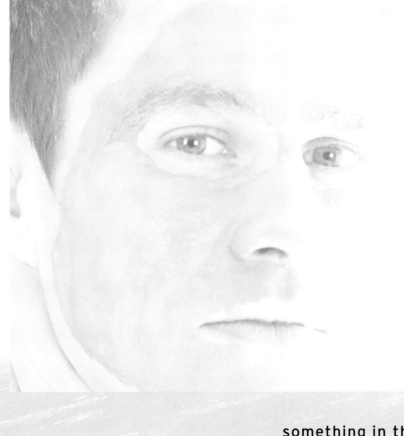

something in the air

One of the best ways to hydrate your skin is to maintain humidity in the

atmosphere. In centrally heated homes and offices or during dry summers,

boost moisture levels and add an element of feng shui, with a dish of scented

water (just add a few drops of a favorite essential oil), a bowl of floating

candles, a pebble fountain, or a trough of water beneath pot plants.

water

cleansing

Water brings new life to whatever has become dusty, tired, and stale. A shower of rain can **refresh** even a busy city street, washing away the detritus of the day. Water can do the same for us. As it strips away the grime and sweat that build up during the day, removes harmful bacteria and viruses, and also stimulates the circulation, water leaves no trace behind but the fresh **natural** scent of clean skin.

water

from the sea

Not surprisingly, bathing can help you to detox (remove harmful toxins from your body), at least from the outside. Salt and seaweed baths have a diuretic effect, which helps flush waste from the body and tone it, if only temporarily.

a salt bath

Epsom salts, made from magnesium sulphate, are a traditional treatment that draws acidic wastes from the body. They also improve circulation and soothe aching joints. Pour a large handful of Epsom salts into a comfortably warm bath and soak for five minutes—you should feel the warmth spreading throughout your body—then massage yourself with a loofah or bath mitt, working toward the heart. This bath can be quite enervating so it is best taken at the end of the day or before a period of relaxation. Avoid this

soothing salt bath if you have high

blood pressure, heart or kidney

problems or cuts and grazes,

which will sting.

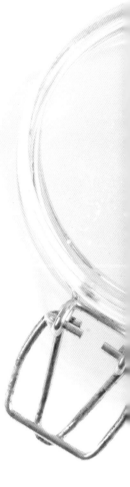

seaweed treatments

Thalassotherapy (seawater treatment) is especially popular in France, where there are now more than 40 coastal centers. They are similar to inland spas except that they use sea water rather than water from thermal springs. Sea water contains large quantities of minerals and trace elements that can aid elimination. Seaweed, an essential part of thalassotherapy, contains them too, but in greater concentrations. Seaweed is also said to have an affinity with blood plasma that enables minerals and trace elements to be absorbed easily through the skin.

bringing it home

Health spas and beauty clinics offer seaweed wraps to encourage inch loss, but you can enjoy its benefits at home with seaweed powder, cream, or salts. If you have very dry skin, there is evidence to show that Dead Sea products—from a sea that has an amazingly high concentration of salt—can be very helpful. You can buy them as soaps or powders, or as a cream that makes your skin as slippery as a seal—but leaves it feeling wonderfully moist and smooth.

water

sweating it out

Steam or Turkish baths help remove toxins by encouraging perspiration (when we are ill, the body often sweats to remove harmful bugs). The heat increases blood circulation just underneath the skin and stimulates the sweat glands. Spas sometimes add essential oil of lavender to the steam to make this a much more sensuous experience. The heat and moisture of the bath can also help relax the muscles and ease aches and pains.

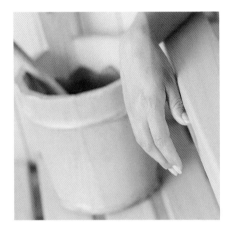

Saunas work in much the same way but minus the steam. A sauna should not be completely dry, though—water and ladles are provided to humidify the atmosphere and, traditionally, birch twigs are provided to stimulate the circulation. Because of the heat, saunas and steam baths are not recommended for pregnant women or anyone with low or high blood pressure or a heart condition.

Five to ten minutes at a time is long enough to enjoy the benefits of a steam bath or sauna, though you can return to it two or three times with breaks in between. Drink plenty of water afterward to make up for the fluids lost through perspiration. Follow your session with a cold shower or dip in a plunge pool to get your circulation going. You will feel refreshed, relaxed, and energized.

water

skin brushing

Exfoliate your body, improve blood circulation and lymph flow, and encourage the production of sebum, the body's

natural moisturizer, with this simple but effective routine.

Ideally do this before having a bath or shower, because you can wash away the skin debris afterward. Use a very soft bristle brush—a baby's hairbrush will do—or a dry face cloth. If you opt for a loofah, wield it with care, and change to a cloth for sensitive areas like the stomach. Before brushing, make sure your skin is completely dry. Start at your feet and work upward with long, firm strokes in sections, from ankle to knee and knee to waist. Then, brush your chest (avoiding the nipples) and back, and your arms, starting with the hands.

As with all forms of massage, follow the veins by working toward the heart.

Avoid brushing your face. Brush your abdomen clockwise—to be more in tune with the flow of blood and the working of the abdomen.

what is lymph?

Lymph is a clear fluid that circulates through your body, carrying away toxins and distributing disease-fighting white blood cells. The fluid drains into lymph nodes (glands), where it is filtered, trapping harmful organisms. The lymph nodes become swollen when coping with infection; that is why you can often feel the nodes in your neck ("swollen glands") when you have a throat infection.

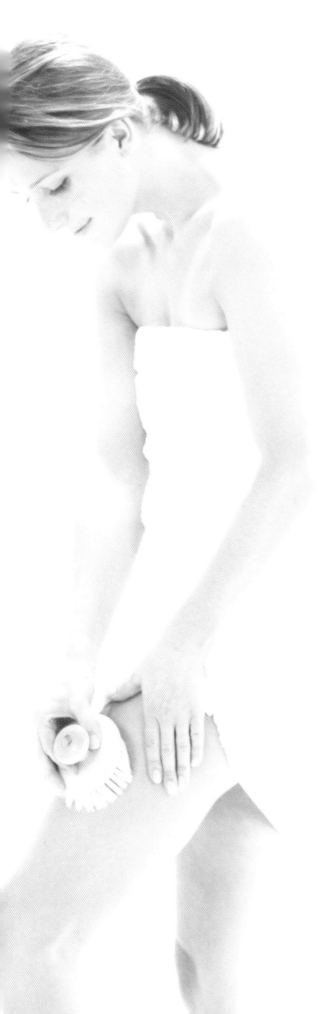

Follow skin brushing with a bath or shower, ending

with a half-a-minute drench with cold water. If you

prefer, decrease the temperature gradually, from

warm to tepid, cool, and then cold. Finish by rubbing

yourself briskly with a towel to warm up again.

water

peach or orange?

Cellulite—is it where toxins collect, lack of elasticity, or just female fat? Doctors dismiss the idea that there is anything special about cellulite, while those with a more holistic approach regard it as a sign that your body is badly polluted and its natural ecology under threat. Either way, it does not stop women agonizing over the orange-peel skin that collects on the bottom, thighs, and sometimes the tops of the arms.

So what to do? A whole-body approach, based on a combination of exercise, diet, and massage seems to be the best way to restore your skin to its original peachy smoothness. Exercise strengthens the muscles and tones the skin, diet reduces fat, and regular massage stimulates the blood supply to all areas of the body. Working together, they should vastly improve the look and texture of your skin in just a few months.

the action plan

Concentrate on exercises to tone specific areas—leg lifts and curls to firm the buttocks, stretches for the inner thighs, weights for the upper arms.

Lose weight, if you need to, following a diet based on fruits and vegetables rather than protein and carbohydrate, and drinking four pints of water a day.

Finally, massage the cellulite skin regularly with a sponge or mitt. You can rub in anticellulite creams containing horse chestnut and ivy, which are designed to boost circulation and remove toxins, or use a couple of drops of energizing rosemary and cleansing fennel essential oils in a few tablespoons of a neutral base oil, such as sweet almond.

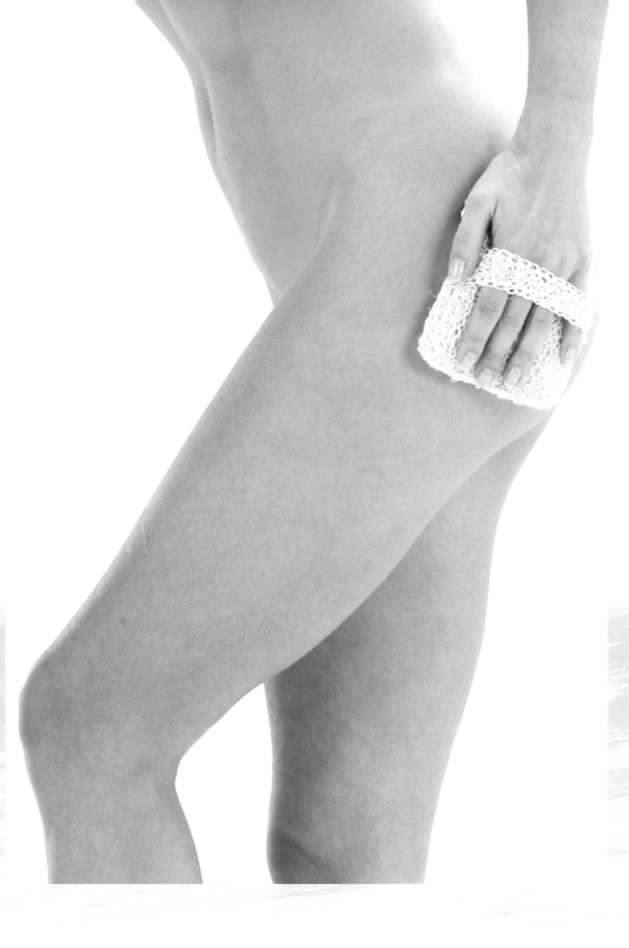

water

the detox dilemma

time for a change

Detox is a beauty buzzword, especially after holidays, when seasonal excess makes the idea of mortifying the flesh, just a little, seem appealing. But what exactly does it mean to detox? Deconstructed, it is simply shorthand for deep cleansing, speeding the removal of wastes and toxins from the body.

The body has its own effective methods of waste disposal, and obsessive detoxing, especially when constant purging and fasting are involved, is mentally unhealthy and can be physically harmful. On the other hand, weeks of eating a diet of high-fat, highly processed foods full of additives, too little exercise, and too much alcohol, can leave your system crying out for a rest. So should you detox? The answer is yes—but not to extremes. Starvation diets and lengthy detox programs can be hell and are not necessary. A couple of days of stripped-down, eating, that kick start a balanced, healthy diet though, could work wonders.

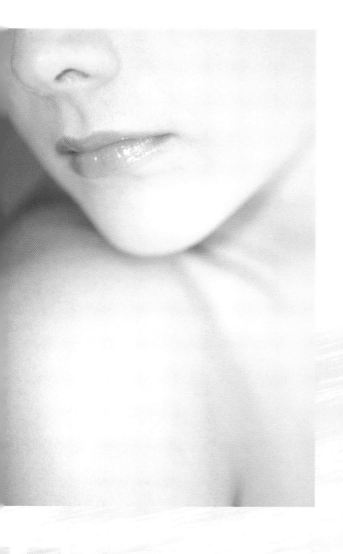

gut instinct

Does the colon need cleansing? The colon is not always the

smooth, self-cleansing organism it should be. Diverticular

disease, thought to result from years of eating refined,

low-fiber foods, now affects the majority of people over 50 in

the West. It starts when undigested matter collects in

pouches in the gut wall and can cause infection (diverticulitis)

as well as pain. But enemas, colonic irrigation, and laxatives,

are crude and potentially hazardous ways of shifting internal

waste. Better to cleanse the system by drinking water, and to

try a diet high in fruits and vegetables.

lemma

water

when to detox

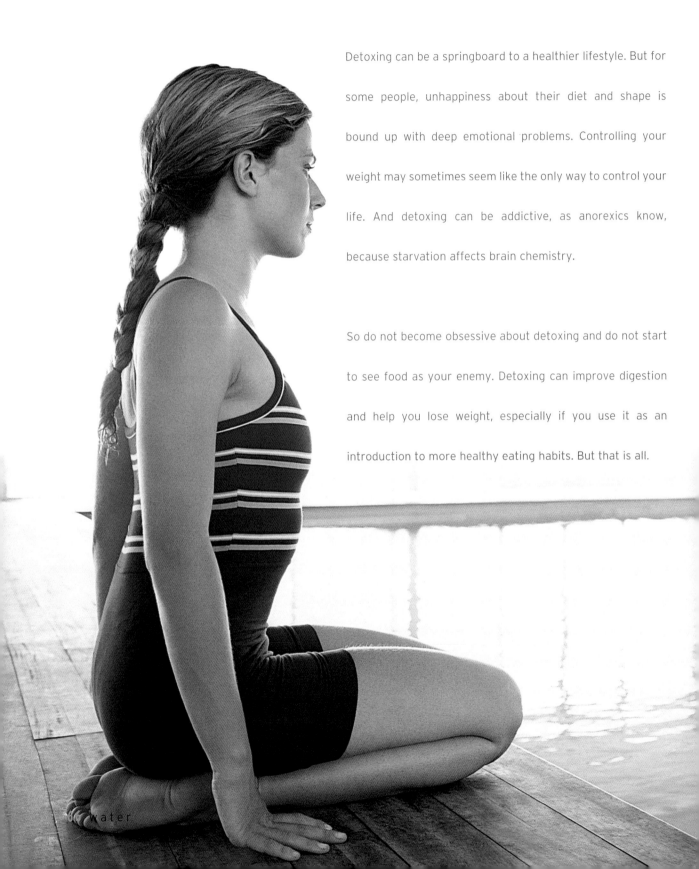

Detoxing can be a springboard to a healthier lifestyle. But for some people, unhappiness about their diet and shape is bound up with deep emotional problems. Controlling your weight may sometimes seem like the only way to control your life. And detoxing can be addictive, as anorexics know, because starvation affects brain chemistry.

So do not become obsessive about detoxing and do not start to see food as your enemy. Detoxing can improve digestion and help you lose weight, especially if you use it as an introduction to more healthy eating habits. But that is all.

detox when...

You cannot face another chocolate.

You have a hangover every weekend (or conversely, your
consumption has increased and you only get a hangover after a
major binge—which is a sign that your body is trying to cope
with your intake and also a step on the way to dependency).

You are putting on weight because you have been eating
unhealthily and need to kick-start a change in your lifestyle.

do **not** detox if...

You are depressed.

You loathe the way you look.

You feel a change of shape will help solve problems with
relationships.

You are ill or recovering from a virus.

water

how to detox

set your own pace

You do not have to starve to detox: Simply drinking four pints of water a day will start the process, flushing the kidneys, easing the passage of waste through the colon and clearing your skin.

If you want to go a step further, try a brief detox diet. Do not go to extremes: A day is good to start with, and three days is probably enough. It is better to incorporate some of the healthy living principles into your everyday life than to follow a punishing regime for a week every few months.

Choose a program that is realistic for you. Since one aim of detoxing is to give your liver a break, you could start by simply avoiding alcohol and rich food. Three days without caffeine (coffee, tea, cola, and chocolate) and processed foods would also be beneficial. And if you want to go further, cutting out dairy foods (milk, yogurt, cheese), wheat, meat, and fish—though there is nothing wrong with these foods in themselves—will automatically increase the emphasis on fruits and vegetables, rice, oats, and pulses. Wash them down with plenty of water and herbal teas to help your digestive system deal with your increased

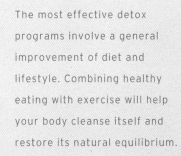

The most effective detox programs involve a general improvement of diet and lifestyle. Combining healthy eating with exercise will help your body cleanse itself and restore its natural equilibrium.

intake of fiber. Do not be surprised if the detox diet

actually makes you feel worse before you feel better.

Some people experience headache, nausea, and

lethargy while following a detox program, though

these symptoms are more likely to occur during

strenuous self-denial. Take it gently.

water

your three day detox plan

Try this whenever you want your diet to become part of the solution rather than part of the problem.

get ready

If you normally take a lot of caffeine and you are planning to cut it out, reduce your intake gradually in the days before your detox—otherwise you will feel irritable and get headaches, which will decrease your chances of completing the plan successfully. Plan three quiet days for your detox, as you will need plenty of rest.

fruits

On the first day, eat fresh fruits only. Fruits contain potassium and are diuretic and mildly laxative. If you feel you need to "fill up," eat plenty of bananas and apples.

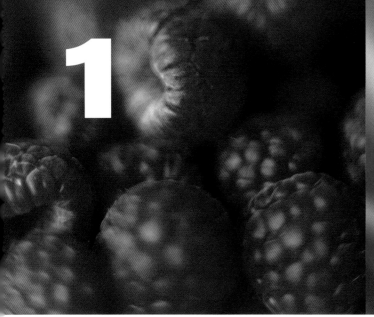

variety

On day two, continue to eat plenty of fruits. Add steamed or raw organic vegetables for your midday and evening meals. Make sure that you are also drinking lots of water.

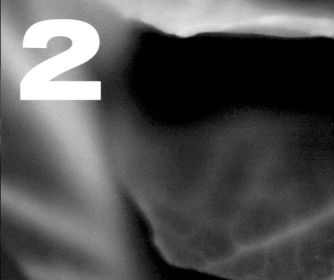

antioxidants

Highly colored fruits like oranges, mango, star fruit, kiwi, and blueberries are rich in antioxidant vitamins thought to protect against cancer and heart disease. If you hanker after starch, try bananas to boost your levels of serotonin, the feel-good hormone in the brain, and apples, which are high in fiber. Pineapple and papaya both contain enzymes (bromelain in pineapple, papain in papaya) that help break down protein and aid digestion.

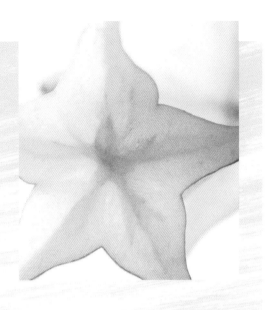

variety

On day three, build on to your existing diet with organic salads, pulses, and gluten-free grains (brown rice, barley, and sweet corn). Avoid bulking up on bread and other gluten-rich products.

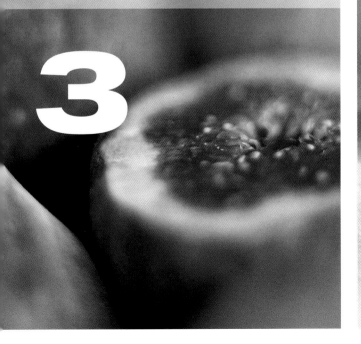

3

slowly

After the three days have passed, return gradually to your normal eating pattern, reintroducing wheat, dairy foods, meat, and fish one by one, and excluding caffeine and alcohol until the end of the week.

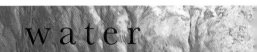

water

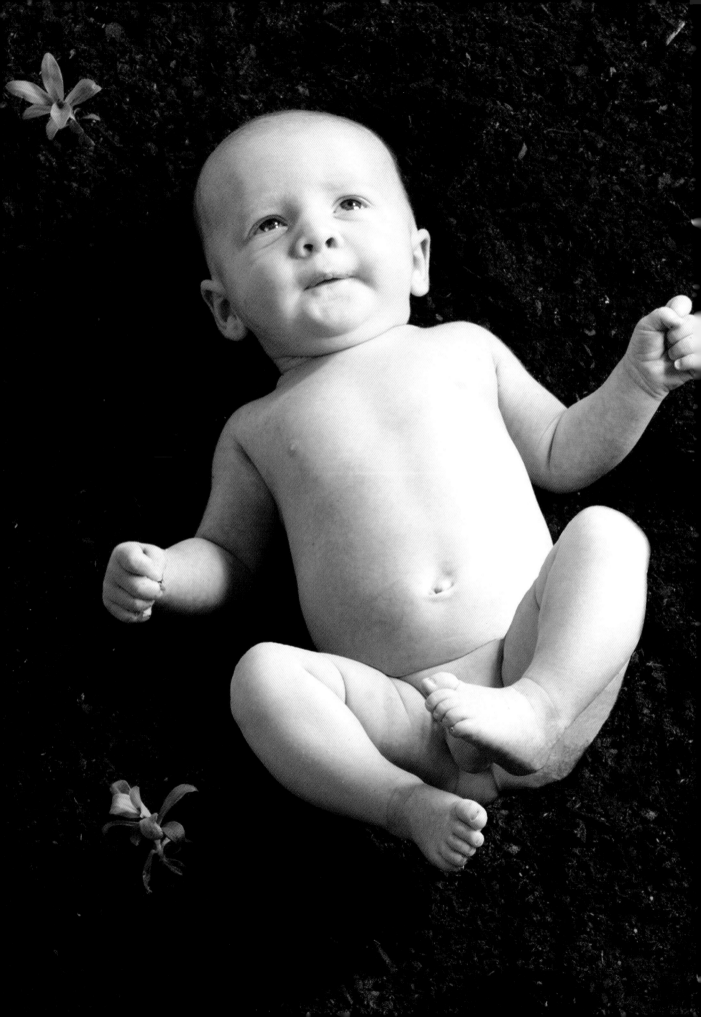

earth

Earth is a storehouse of unrivalled
richness and variety. Out of the brown
earth rises the harvest of fruits, leaves,
and grains that are the staples of the
human diet, along with the grass essential
for milk and meat. Earth nurtures us in
other ways too, because deep beneath
the surface lie the minerals that power
industry and provide material wealth.
Earth is the fertile red clay that gave
rise to Adam, the first man.

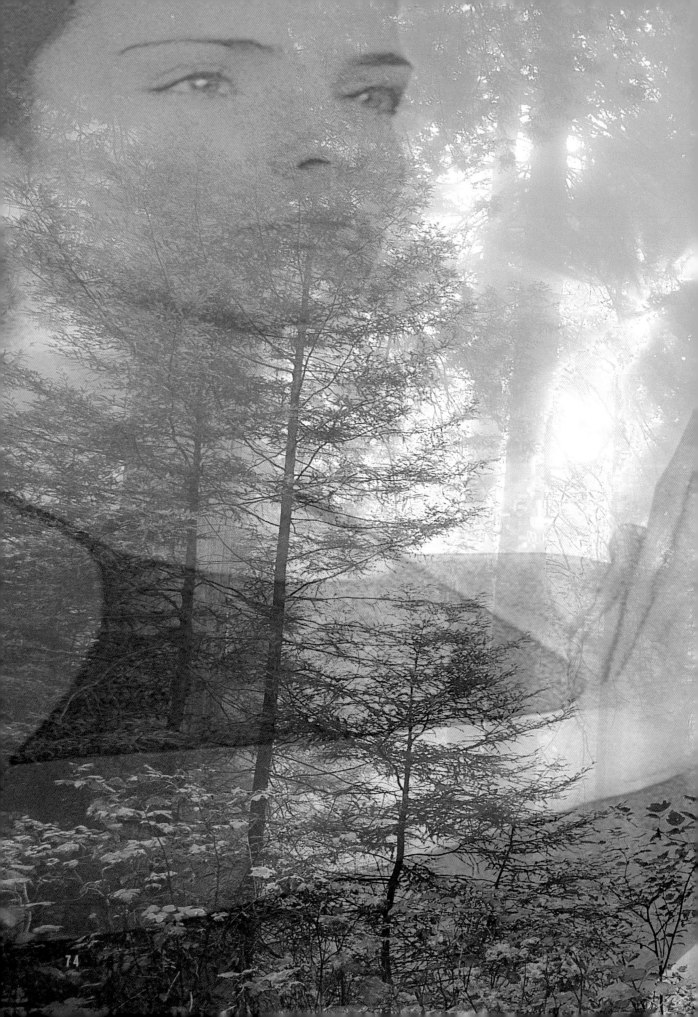

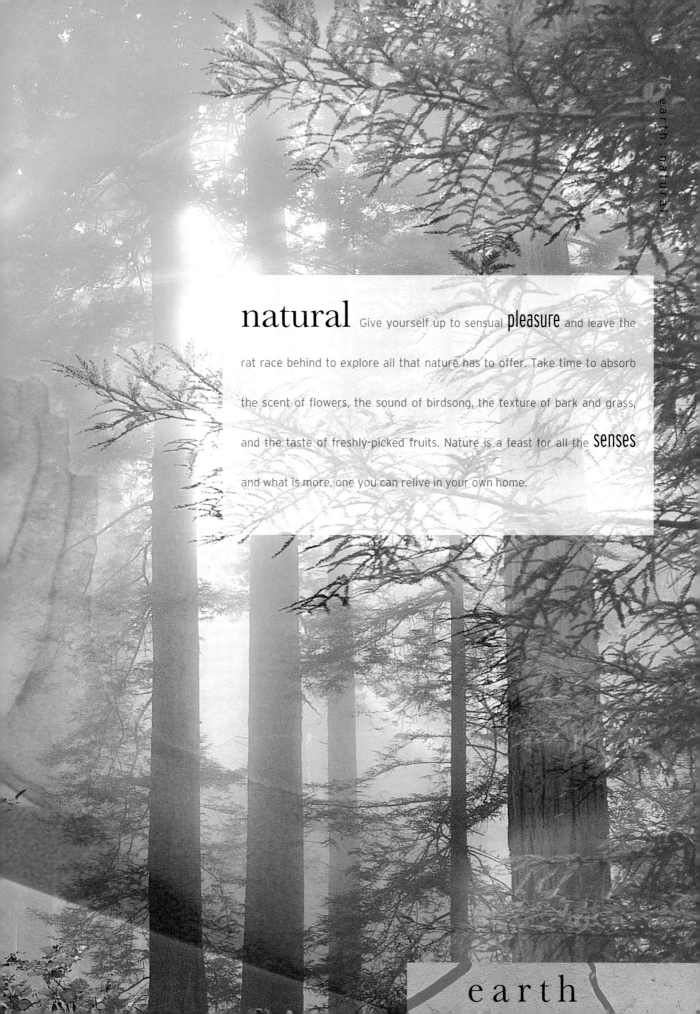

natural

Give yourself up to sensual **pleasure** and leave the rat race behind to explore all that nature has to offer. Take time to absorb the scent of flowers, the sound of birdsong, the texture of bark and grass, and the taste of freshly-picked fruits. Nature is a feast for all the **senses** and what is more, one you can relive in your own home.

earth

the naked face

It is hard to beat natural goodness. A close look at skin care ranges shows that despite an impressively scientific contents list, most rely on familiar plants and foods for their principal active ingredients. Pick up a moisturizer and you may well find it contains AHAs—alpha-hydroxy acids, commonly known as fruit acids, but which include lactic acid from milk products, too.

Natural ingredients in popular beauty products range from the everyday to the exotic—think of milk bath, cucumber foot lotion, tea tree and mint bodywash, clove shampoo....What is more questionable is how much of the plant they actually contain, and whether it is a natural essence or a synthesized version developed in a laboratory.

the skin vitamin

The strongest peeling action of all, so much so that some versions are available only on prescription, belongs to vitamin A which, as retinol and retinoic acid, is found in antiaging creams and treatments for acne. Turn to creams for dry skin and you will find vitamin E, known for its regenerating quality, while GLA (gamma linolenic acid) from evening primrose and borage oils, which has a soothing anti-inflammatory action, appears in skin-care ranges for sensitive skin.

Using individual ingredients to make up your own "simples" (as homemade unguents and remedies were once called) allows you to draw on the full potency of the plants you choose. Not all the cosmetics you make will be as consistent as those available in the shops and you may need to keep masks in place with a fine layer of cheesecloth. Fresh cosmetics do not contain preservatives, so all, except oils, need to be made in small quantities and stored in the refrigerator. But they are easy to put together and surprisingly effective.

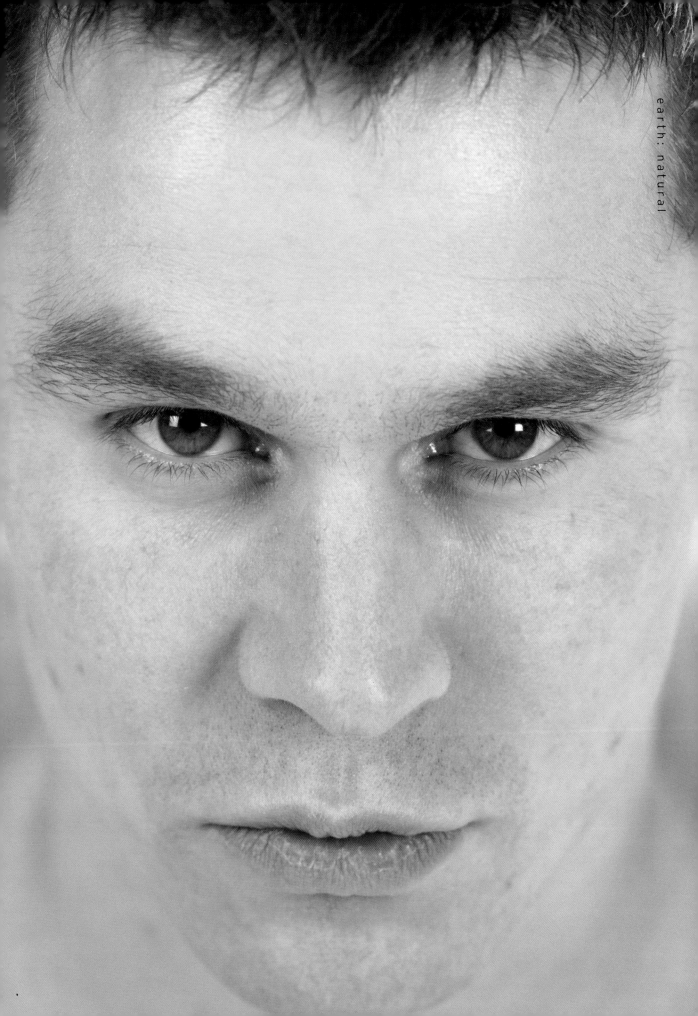

simples for dry skin

Pamper parched skin with natural oils and essences.

egg and honey mask

Eggs yield protein while honey helps to moisturize.

Beat a medium egg yolk and mix with two teaspoons of

honey. Slather on to face and neck, avoiding the eyes,

and leave for ten minutes before rinsing off.

orange and rosewater toner

Blend two fragrant waters to make this soothing toner. Take two tablespoons each of orange flower water, rosewater, and still spring water and add to a jar with a teaspoon of glycerin. Shake vigorously.

coconut cream cleanser

For an instant cleanser that is a luxurious alternative to mineral oils, use coconut cream, a staple of Indian cooking. Dip cotton wool balls and apply to the skin, working upward with gentle, circular movements.

Any ingredient can cause a sensitivity reaction, so always try a little first on an inconspicuous place, like the inside of the elbow, and wait for 24 hours before proceeding.

earth

simples for sensitive skin

At its best, skin is delicately translucent; on a bad skin day, it can be flaky, patchy, and irritable. Here are some natural remedies to improve your skin and help keep it feeling soft and bright.

milk and chamomile cleanser

It could not be simpler: Just add three tablespoons of fresh chamomile heads (half that amount of dried) to half a pint of full cream milk and leave to soak for an hour. Warm gently in a saucepan over a low heat, then strain before applying to the skin.

carrot balm

This balm is perfect for calming troubled skin. Grate an organic carrot into a pot of natural yogurt and leave the mixture in the refrigerator for several hours. Strain before applying to the skin.

peach toner

The anti-inflammatory action of peach juice is ideal for sensitive skins. Squeeze the juice from a large peach, strain, and mix with equal parts of still spring water.

marigold rinse

With its antiseptic and antifungal properties, the pot marigold (calendula) is one of the staples of the traditional herb garden, famous for its ability to soothe sore skin. Pour a pint of freshly boiled water over four ounces of fresh marigold heads (half that amount of dried) and leave until cool. Strain the rinse before use.

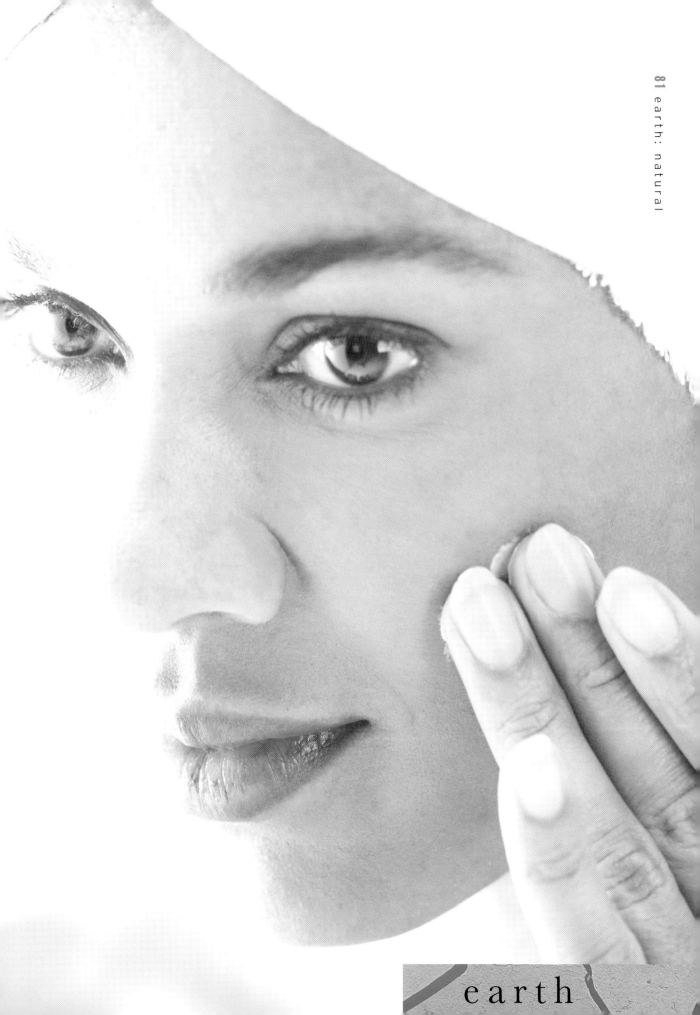

earth

simples for oily skin

It may be shiny and spot-prone now, but because it retains its bloom and contours longer than other types, you will

bless it later. Follow these tips for natural control over oily skin.

egg white mask

This is a quick way to remove excess oil. Separate an

egg and whisk the white. Spread it over neck, face

(avoiding the eyes), and upper back and leave until

dry. Beat the yolk and leave for ten minutes, then use

it to rinse off the egg white, followed by a water rinse.

cabbage lotion

This is an anti-inflammatory rinse that is excellent for keeping spots at bay. Strip half a pound of cabbage leaves from the stalk and ribs and liquefy in a blender. Mix with half a pint of distilled witch hazel and half a teaspoon of lemon juice, then strain. Apply to the T-zone twice a day to help keep your skin blemish-free.

lavender rinse

Lavender is a natural antiseptic, ideal for treating skin that has a tendency to break out. Pour a pint of freshly boiled water over 14 ounces of dried lavender flowers, then leave to cool and strain. Apply twice daily. Treat spots with essential oil of lavender applied neat.

earth

simples for normal skin

If you don't have to think too hard about skin care, the chances are that your skin is normal—not too dry, too oily, or too sensitive. These natural remedies will help keep it that way.

lemon bleach for hands & arms

This combination will provide a quick fix for dull skin. Take the squeezed halves of two lemons. Add a little olive oil to two of them and rest your elbows in them for 15 minutes. Meanwhile, use the remaining lemon halves on your nails, cuticles, and any discolored areas on your skin such as liver spots, then dunk your nails in olive oil for ten minutes. Afterward, rinse, pat dry, and slather on hand or body cream.

yogurt mask

This soothing mask is good for most skins. Mix a teaspoonful of liquid honey with a tablespoonful of natural yogurt. Apply to face and neck, avoiding the eyes, and leave for ten minutes.

cucumber lotion

Refreshing and brightening, cucumber has a mild bleaching action and is said to combat wrinkles too. Liquefy half a cucumber and strain off the juice. Mix with equal parts of rosewater and enough glycerin to give consistency. Use as a hand lotion or facial wash.

strawberry skin tonic

To brighten sallow or dull skin, liquefy half a dozen fresh, ripe strawberries and add to a quarter pint of full cream milk (test for sensitivity first). Pat the mixture onto your skin and leave for a few minutes before rinsing off.

marigold and yogurt cleanser

This refreshing cleanser contains soothing marigold to cosset the skin. Take two

tablespoonfuls of fresh pot marigold heads and pour over a quarter pint of freshly

boiled water. Leave to cool before straining, then mix with a pot of natural yogurt.

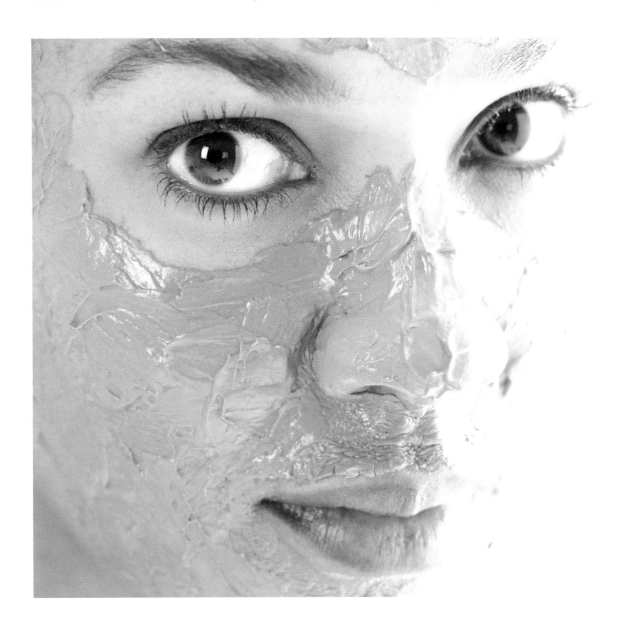

earth

simples for mature skin

Finer, dryer, less elastic skin (hence wrinkles) needs cosseting with the richest ingredients nature can provide.

rose, clary, and vitamin E oil

This provides a beautifully fragrant way to nourish the skin. Pierce a natural-source vitamin E capsule and take two drops, then mix with three drops each of rose and clary essential oils in two tablespoons of sweet almond or apricot oil. Store any remaining oil straight away in a dark glass bottle with a tight stopper and keep in a cool place. Apply the oil at bedtime, preferably after a warm bath. Leave for half an hour and tissue away the excess.

three-oil antiaging treatment

This is a simple remedy, yet one of the best. Blend two tablespoons each of apricot, sweet almond, and wheat germ oil and keep in an opaque, sealed container. Use on the forehead and around the eyes and mouth to minimize wrinkles.

herbal eye balm

Ten minutes is all you need to revive tired eyes and reduce dark circles. Soak two chamomile tea bags in a little freshly boiled water and then put in the refrigerator. While they are cooling, peel and slice a potato. Lie down with the potato slices over your eyes and the tea bags resting on the potato slices.

banana face mask

This is an easy way to plump out wrinkles. Mash half a

small banana until smooth and lump-free, then apply

to the face. Leave for 15 minutes before rinsing clean.

carrot toner

Carrots have a moisturizing effect that helps soothe

dry skin and are rich in vitamin A, used in retinol

creams to reduce the signs of aging. For this simple,

extract the juice from four large carrots. Strain and

dilute the juice with an equal amount of still spring

water. (Test for sensitivity first.)

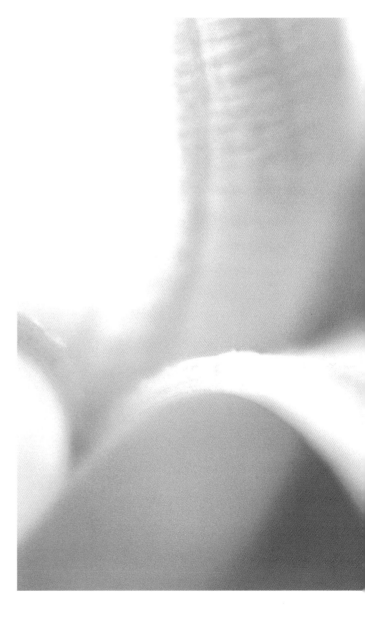

earth

hair simples

From vinegar rinses that add shine to dark hair to beer for extra body, natural hair treatments have a long pedigree. Here are a few you may not know.

hair rescue

For damaged hair. Pour two tablespoons of olive oil into an eggcup and warm in a pan of hot water. Work the oil through the hair, then pile your hair on top of your head and cover with cellophane wrap, topped with a hot, damp towel. Leave for up to an hour. Wash your hair with mild shampoo.

three-fruit hair reviver

In a blender, mix together a small banana with two heaped tablespoons of avocado and two of melon, one tablespoon of sunflower oil and one of plain yogurt. Work into the hair from the roots to the tips and leave for 15 minutes before shampooing.

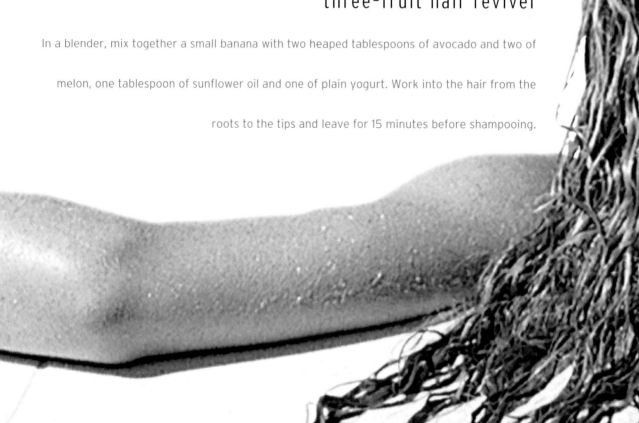

henna hair reviver

Henna adds a gloss that suits any natural hair type. Take one pack of neutral henna and mix to a paste with cool water. Add a beaten egg yolk and a tablespoonful of milk, then comb through the hair. Leave for an hour before shampooing.

perfect shampoo

Make a herbal infusion using four tablespoons of fresh herbs (or two of dried). Choose calendula or marshmallow, plus a little sweet almond oil for dry hair, calendula or lavender for processed hair, and rosemary or sage to add shine. Strain and mix with three tablespoons of baby shampoo and add a few drops of matching essential oil for extra fragrance.

earth

mud, glorious mud

The Neydharting Moor spa in Austria uses one of the most popular treatments in the world: Mud. Once only available to patrons of the Grosspertholtz Clinic, the mud is now available in a variety of products from body masks to drinks. What makes it so special and so sought after is its organic richness. For thousands of years, myriads of plants and animals have sunk into its waters, creating a black mud dense in nutrients that not only soften the skin but are thought to relieve a variety of physical complaints from joint pains to gastric ulcers. Neyharting Moor is not the only source of health-giving mud, though with a pedigree that goes back almost 300 years, it is one of the oldest. Native Americans also used therapeutic mud, and recently a new moor has been discovered near Quebec in Canada with similar properties to Neyharting. The sea hides similar riches, and mud from the Dead Sea is also known for its unique properties, especially

recommended for dry skin, eczema, and psoriasis. So

much moisture is lost through evaporation there that

the mud contains a high concentration of minerals

and salts of magnesium, sodium, calcium,

and potassium.

earth

have a wallow

A mud bath is the easiest way to access these health and beauty benefits. For the full therapeutic effect, a 20-minute mud bath every other day for 42 days is recommended—in theory you shouldn't shower afterward if you want to gain the full benefit, because it continues to act for a further 24 hours. The second method is to use a body mask, applied in much the same way as a face mask. Turn up the thermostat so the air temperature is warm enough for you to lie naked, then make yourself comfortable on a sheet or

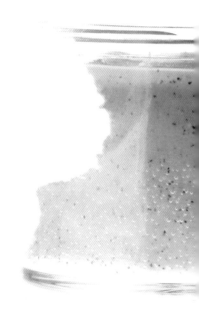

93 earth: natural

in a dry bath. The mud is painted on (enlist the help of a partner if you can) and kept in place for the recommended time before being washed away, leaving the skin smooth and soft. The mask contains all of the beneficial ingredients of the fresh mud.

Or take your mud therapy one step further, with a do-it-yourself body wrap, covering your whole body except for the head, hands, and feet, in the thick black mud. Wrap yourself in warm towels and leave the mud for half an hour before showering, so that the active ingredients can get to work. Moor mud and Dead Sea products for home use can be bought from beauty spas or on-line. You could also treat yourself to a trip to a beauty salon, where you can sample the more complex treatments based on clay, especially sea clay. You could seek out Ionotherapy, for example, which combines electrical treatment with a clay and textile wrap, and is said to create instant inch loss.

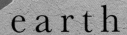

earth

get stoned

Another popular "earth" treatment is LaStone therapy, developed by masseuse Mary Nelson-Hannigan from Native American treatments using basalt (hot) and marble (cold) rocks. Like body wraps, the method uses heat to relax the muscles, but it also aims to induce a state of deep meditation. Protected by a sheet, you lie back on two rows of warmed stones. Large stones are placed on the belly and chest, small ones between your toes; you are then massaged with a warm rock. A bit ambitious to try at home? Maybe, but it is easy to combine warmed stone treatment with reflexology, which concentrates on your feet but invigorates your whole body.

warmed stone therapy

Warm a selection of smooth, round pebbles (from the seashore or a garden

center) on a radiator, or soak in boiling water and then dry thoroughly.

Wash your feet and sprinkle with corn flour or starch-based talc. Place the

warmed stones between your toes to stimulate the acupressure points.

When your feet feel completely relaxed, treat them one at a time. Lay one

foot across your knee and massage it thoroughly, starting at the ankle.

Now "walk" the top of your thumb slowly across the area you want to treat

a few times, then grasp your foot and rotate it from the ankle, pressing the

thumb into the spot. (The right foot corresponds to the right side of the

body, the left to the left.)

For tension in the shoulders and upper back, work the area beneath the little toe where the foot widens.

For cystitis and kidney problems, treat the sensitive inside of the foot in an area extending from the heel into the arch of the foot.

Long-term biliousness and overindulgence can have a detrimental effect on the liver. Treat this by massaging the entire arch of the foot, starting from the outside of the heel.

For indigestion, walk your thumbs just below the ball of the foot, from the inside of the foot across the arch.

Massage the center of the second and third toes to relieve eye strain and headaches behind the eyes.

To treat backache and stiffness, massage the inside rim of the foot from top to bottom.

For insomnia and anxiety, rotate your thumb at a central point just below the ball of the foot, then lower down, about an inch toward the inside of the foot. Finally, massage the fleshy pads of the big toes, concentrating on the centers.

Headache and sinus pain can be treated by massaging the outer edge of the big toe.

Tension often originates in the neck. Work the "neck" of the big toe, just above the ball of the foot.

Rub each of the toes, concentrating just below the tips, to ease colds and catarrh.

earth

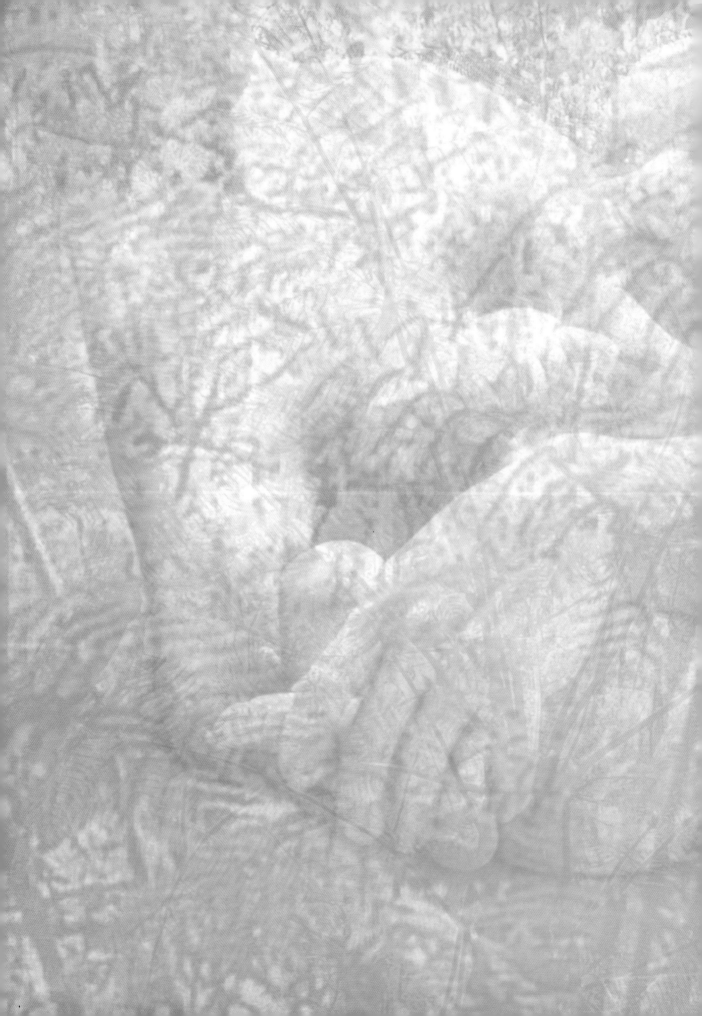

nurturing

Simple foods, beautifully prepared, are not just for gourmets. They keep the body in peak condition, with **glowing** skin, shiny hair, strong bones and muscles, and an active brain. Food provides the energy required to enjoy life to the full and helps build immunity to combat disease. Indeed, food is so **powerful**, it can even improve your mind.

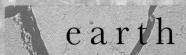

earth

the naked diet

In the first months of life, a single food is all the nourishment you need, sustaining the growth that occurs as body weight doubles and new brain connections are forged. When milk alone is no longer enough, new tastes are introduced slowly, with the accent on foods rich in vitamins and free from additives. But fast-forward 20 years and what do you find? A diet that draws on a tremendous variety of foods, all too often intensively farmed, highly processed and low in nutrient value.

Time then to return to a simple way of eating. It can be difficult to change the eating habits of a lifetime. Palates attuned to high-fat, high-salt and highly flavored foods, sweets, and chocolate can reject a switch to more natural foods, which seem bland until your taste buds become aware of the subtleties. So why not try this?

For a week, eat anything you like, apart from processed foods. Fresh, organic foods in season should be your first choice but prepared and frozen are acceptable. Steam vegetables lightly or eat them raw, and if you eat meat and fish, choose free-range, not factory-farmed, varieties. Ready-meals, ready-made pastries, sausages, ham, and smoked fish are out, cookies and cakes should be home-baked and, ideally, even bread should be home-baked. Without any effort, you should find yourself eating the nutrient-dense diet that experts recommend; rich in complex carbohydrates for sustained energy, high in fiber, and low in fat, salt, and sugar. By the end of the

week, you should begin to appreciate the fresh, natural

taste of good food. What is more, if you struggle to keep

in shape, you are almost guaranteed to lose weight—

pastries and cakes are far less tempting when you're

faced with preparing them yourself.

Returning to a simpler way of eating is not only a recipe for

good health, but a reminder of how sensuous eating can be.

Foods eaten at their peak is an unforgettable experience.

Proust, famously, remembered the madeleines; your

equivalent might be the sweetness of ripe strawberries or

bread hot from the oven. Because taste is associated with

parts of the brain dealing with emotions and memory, the

aroma of food can take you straight back into the past.

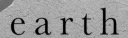

earth

eat well, be well

A piece of fruit changed Eve's life, and it could do the same for yours. Just eating an extra two or three ounces of fruits (or vegetables—take your pick) every day reduces the chances of dying from heart disease by 20 percent, according to a recent study of almost 20,000 people. Those with the highest intake of vitamin C had the most protection, regardless of whether they smoked or had high blood pressure, both risk factors for heart disease.

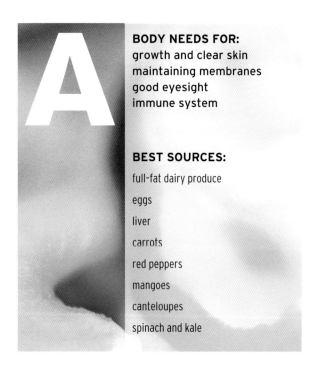

A

BODY NEEDS FOR:
growth and clear skin
maintaining membranes
good eyesight
immune system

BEST SOURCES:
full-fat dairy produce
eggs
liver
carrots
red peppers
mangoes
canteloupes
spinach and kale

So it really does work—but how? By acting on the immune system, giving the body the strength it needs to ward off disease and offset the impact of stress, pollution, and lack of sleep.

Vitamin C is one of the antioxidants that are among the most powerful allies in the fight against disease. When fats oxidize, they release the harmful free radicals responsible for the cell damage leading to

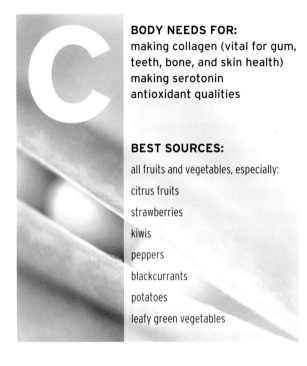

C

BODY NEEDS FOR:
making collagen (vital for gum, teeth, bone, and skin health)
making serotonin
antioxidant qualities

BEST SOURCES:

all fruits and vegetables, especially:

citrus fruits

strawberries

kiwis

peppers

blackcurrants

potatoes

leafy green vegetables

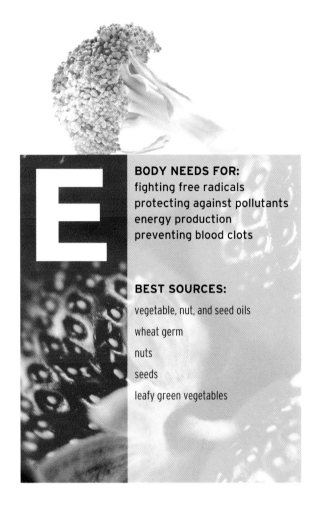

E

BODY NEEDS FOR:
fighting free radicals
protecting against pollutants
energy production
preventing blood clots

BEST SOURCES:

vegetable, nut, and seed oils

wheat germ

nuts

seeds

leafy green vegetables

aging, heart disease, and cancer. Foods rich in the antioxidant vitamins C, E, and beta-carotene (which the body converts to vitamin A) mop up these free radicals. So turn to highly colored fruits and veggies (kiwis, broccoli, oranges, tomatoes) for vitamin C and beta-carotene, wheat germ, sunflower oils, and avocados to top up your supplies of vitamin E. Consuming antioxidants also reduces the risk of developing lung conditions like asthma and bronchitis,

which is one of the reasons why the World Health Organization recommends eating a minimum of five portions—half a pound—of fruits and vegetables a day.

Experts agree it is best to eat natural foods. You may miss out on vital elements if you opt for tablets. There are cases where supplements are recommended. For example, women trying for a baby are encouraged to take supplements of folic acid, one of the B vitamins.

earth

gifts from the soil

Hidden within the earth are the minerals and trace elements that are vital for good health. A surprising number of these—more than a dozen—are considered essential for general health, but only very small quantities are required. You can make the most of them by careful food combining. Tea, coffee, bran, spinach, and rhubarb all contain substances that interfere with absorption and should be eaten separately.

boosting

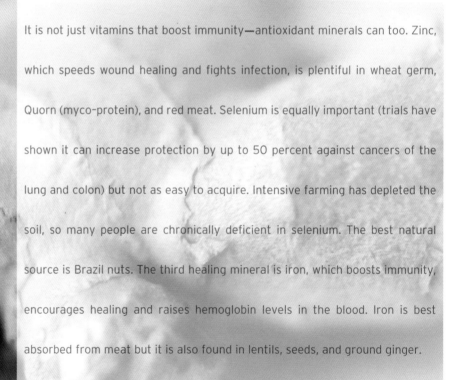

It is not just vitamins that boost immunity—antioxidant minerals can too. Zinc, which speeds wound healing and fights infection, is plentiful in wheat germ, Quorn (myco-protein), and red meat. Selenium is equally important (trials have shown it can increase protection by up to 50 percent against cancers of the lung and colon) but not as easy to acquire. Intensive farming has depleted the soil, so many people are chronically deficient in selenium. The best natural source is Brazil nuts. The third healing mineral is iron, which boosts immunity, encourages healing and raises hemoglobin levels in the blood. Iron is best absorbed from meat but it is also found in lentils, seeds, and ground ginger.

balancing

Foods rich in potassium like bananas, potatoes, and onions help balance the high salt intake that is

a feature of modern diets. Salt, or sodium, is one mineral few people lack and an excess can

contribute to high blood pressure. Reduce your intake by half, using a little less every day so your

palate can adjust, and avoid processed foods, which

often rely on sodium for flavor.

building

Together with vitamin D, calcium and magnesium are essential for strong bones. Fish like sardines are a good way

to absorb both calcium and vitamin D provided you eat the bones, but dairy foods are usually a more convenient

source. (This need not increase your fat intake because low-fat cheese and semi-skimmed milk contain higher

levels than full-fat versions.) Like calcium, magnesium boosts nerve function and muscle power, and helps protect

against heart disease. Top it up with a cup of cocoa:

Made with milk, it is the perfect drink

for bones.

earth

plant alchemy

The most exciting recent discoveries relate to phytochemicals—plant chemicals—that give protection from specific diseases. These mysterious elements cluster in different food groups, traditionally valued for their medicinal and healing powers.

It is allicin, for example, which gives garlic its renowned ability to fight infection, a characteristic that extends to other members of the allium family, such as onions. Garlic has antibacterial properties strong enough to knock out the food-poisoning bacteria salmonella and it is antiviral, too. Together with its antioxidant qualities, these help protect against stomach cancer and ulcers.

Quercetin is an antioxidant found in an abundant range of foods from cabbage, known as the medicine of the poor, to apples, broad beans, black tea, and red wine.

Good for the heart, if bad for the head. Indulging in soft fruits must be one of the most enjoyable ways to protect your health. Ellagic acid—found in cherries, raspberries, and blackberries—is a potent defense against cancer.

But perhaps the most famous functional food is broccoli which, along with sprouts, is rich in cancer-fighting compounds. It is particularly effective for hormonal cancers, thanks to substances called indoles, which have been found to suppress cell activity in breast cancer. So too does lycopene, an antioxidant found in tomatoes, especially cooked tomatoes. Spaghetti sauce, pizza, even ketchup are all good sources that should appeal to men, in more ways than one, because they also help reduce the risk of prostate cancer and heart disease.

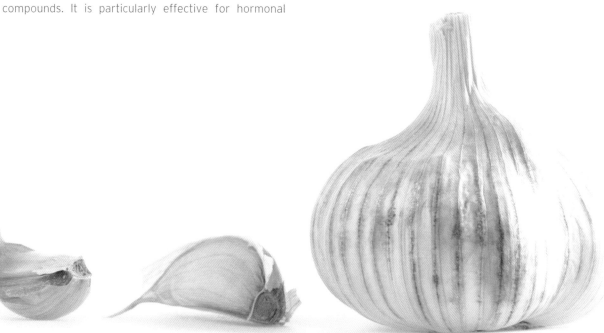

earth

the new food pharmacy

From the exotic to the prosaic, the fruits of the earth are yielding up their secrets. In some cases these are new elements, in others new foods with surprisingly powerful health benefits. Scientists in a range of disciplines are turning their attention to food research. Granted, many of these investigations are new and some may not live up to their early promise, but console yourself with the thought that rarely is the search for knowledge so delicious.

avocado

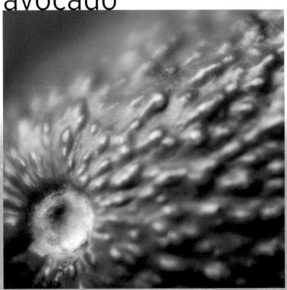

Avocado. Long known as an excellent source of healing vitamin E, avocados have now been found to contain chemicals that protect the liver. A treatment for hepatitis using avocado is being developed.

potatoes

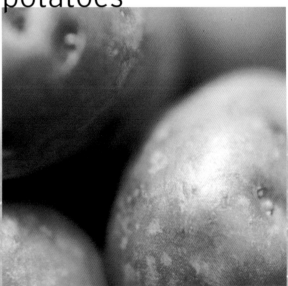

Potatoes. This staple of high-fiber diets may also nourish the brain, according to Canadian research, which found it more effective in boosting memory than the sugar-hit of a high glucose drink.

persimmon

Persimmon. This tomato-like fruit packs twice as much

fiber and a greater concentration of antioxidants than

the average apple into its small size. Make sure your

persimmon is ripe before you eat it.

oolong

Oolong tea. Black and green teas contain antioxidants

that protect against heart disease. Oolong, which is a

blend of both types, has also been shown to soothe

skin complaints like dermatitis.

paw-paw

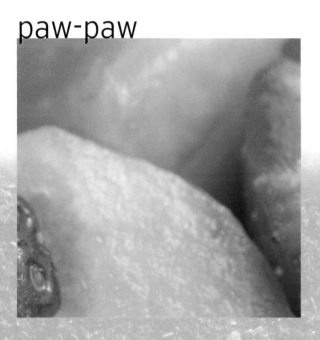

honey

Paw-paw. Scientists are racing to synthesize the

chemicals found in this exotic fruit, which have been

found to destroy cancer cells. In isolation, they are

highly toxic, but you can benefit from their protective

action simply by enjoying the fruit.

Honey. Reputed to be a natural antiseptic that heals

wounds and burns, honey, it seems, is also good for

hangovers. It contains fructose, which competes for

the metabolism of alcohol. So try some toast and

honey the next time you are suffering.

earth

mood foods

Foods provide emotional as well as physical sustenance, but there is real science behind our cravings. They may point to what the body, or the brain, lacks.

happy eating

The compulsion to comfort eat increases with the approach of winter, when lack of sunlight triggers the urge to hibernate. The body cries out for foods that will fuel us through the winter months. In its extreme form, this lethargy, depression, and bingeing on starchy foods becomes what is known as seasonal affective disorder, or SAD. A tendency towards depression and overeating may already be present and SAD merely acts as a trigger, but the evidence in this area is, so far, inconclusive. Most of us experience some emotional response to the coming of winter. There is actually a good reason to eat more carbohydrates when the nights begin to close in and the weather starts getting cold: High-carbohydrate foods help metabolize the amino acid tryptophan, which speeds the release of the feel-good chemical serotonin in the brain. You do not need much, so if you want to avoid the extra weight too many cookies and cakes can pile on, try increasing your intake of bananas, poultry, spinach, and broccoli. These foods are all naturally rich in tryptophan, as well as plenty of other healthy chemicals to help you see the winter in without getting SAD about it. Step up your intake of foods rich in B vitamins too. Found in yeast extract and fortified cereals, the B vitamins can also put you in a better mood.

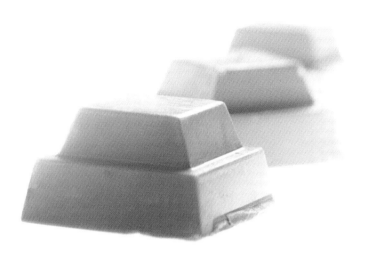

natural high

It is said that 40 percent of women crave chocolate and no wonder: It is virtually psychoactive. For a start, it

contains two powerful stimulants, theobromine (which translated, means food of the gods) and to a lesser extent,

caffeine. It also contains phenylethylamine, which is identical to the chemical released by people in love. It also links

to a brain chemical called dopamine, which can improve concentration and alertness—yet another excuse to eat

chocolate. If you do not want to eat chocolate, try turkey, apples, eggs, and milk instead. You will miss out, though,

on another set of amines found in chocolate. These are chemicals that target the cannabinoid area in the brain,

which is the section that is responsible for creating feelings of euphoria. And that is not all. Although chocolate is

antioxidant, particularly plain chocolate, which contains up to 70 percent cocoa solids and is high in fat, the stearic

acid content of cocoa means that it has a neutral effect on cholesterol levels. On the downside, the feel-good effect

of chocolate is a short-term thing, and bingeing brings its own mental, emotional, and physical problems. Also,

chocolate contains sugar, which will give you a quick high and then bring on a low.

food laid bare

naked vegetables

How would you like a nice dressing with your salad, perhaps made of organophosphates? Unless you go organic, you may not have the choice, because buying pure, uncontaminated food is increasingly difficult. To make sure they are cosmetically acceptable, lettuces are sprayed up to ten times, lemons sealed with wax, and carrots so contaminated, consumers in some countries have been warned to peel them. Meanwhile, according to one recent syrvey, the soil in which fruits and vegetables are grown is leached of goodnes.

As a result, sales of organic foods are booming. Supermarkets are not always the best source, and for food at peak freshness, it is often best to buy direct from the farm or from specialized stores that offer very fresh organic produce. Be prepared to be flexible about what is available, and make sure you wash food thoroughly. For convenience, you can always turn to frozen organics. Frozen food can contain more nutrients and is a better choice by far than tired greens and wrinkled apples.

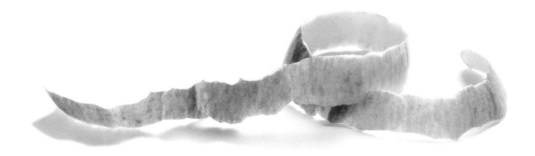

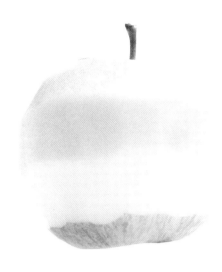

animal rights

Choosing seasonal varieties is another way to buy the best. You cannot always tell just by looking whether an item is truly fresh: Apples, for example, may be stored at carefully regulated temperatures for months before appearing on the shelves and ending up in your fruit bowl. Waiting until fruits and vegetables are in their proper season and are naturally available will reintroduce you to the unsurpassable taste of fresh-picked strawberries, the first sweet-sour apples of fall, or the intense nutty taste of parsnips after a winter frost.

If the impact of intensive farming on fruits and vegetables is alarming, its effect on cattle, poultry, and fish has been catastrophic. Salmonella in eggs and poultry, and parasites in fish are a good argument for turning vegetarian. Even if you don't, self-interest, as well as concern for animal welfare, makes choosing products from animals allowed to roam free and raised on organic feed a priority. Or eat only animals that lived in a natural environment.

earth

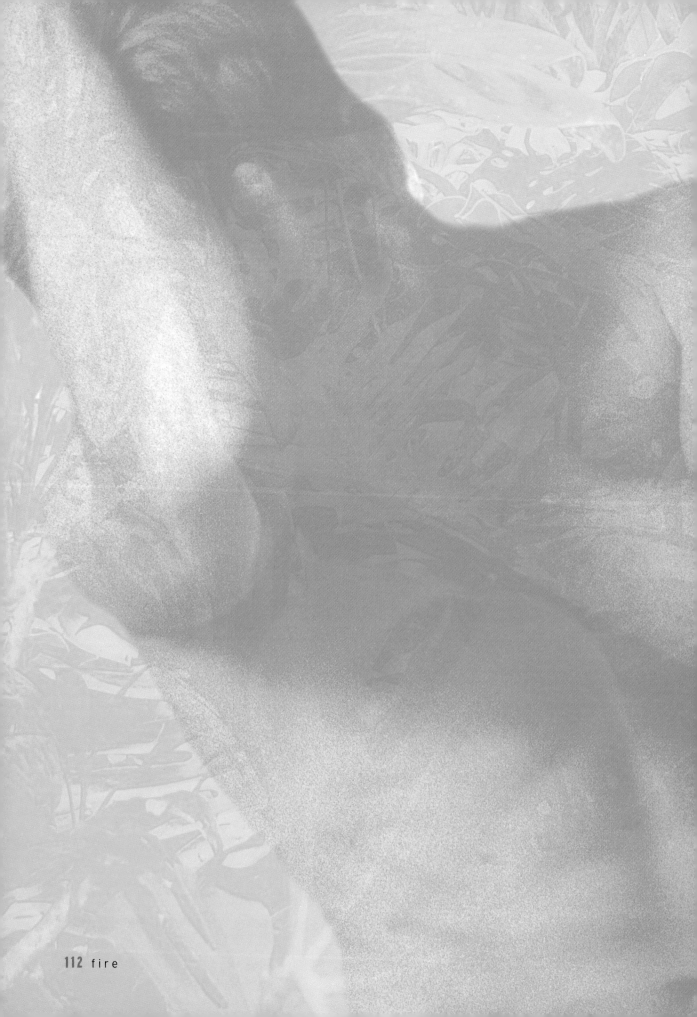

healing

Every year affirms the value of green medicine. Science acknowledges that the most powerful **forces** for healing come from the **earth**, and plants once cultivated by traditional healers are now used to counter the twenty-first-century plagues of heart disease, cancer, and stress. At the same time we are rediscovering the **magic** of touch to stroke away pain, soothe the body, and calm the mind.

earth

living medicine

Step inside any pharmacy and you will see just how much modern medicine owes to traditional herbal cures. Many of today's most important life-saving drugs are originally derived from plants. Two important drugs in the treatment of heart disease are aspirin from meadowsweet and digitalis from foxgloves. The anticarcinogenic drug vincristine is distilled from the African periwinkle, and less than ten years ago Taxol was developed from the Pacific yew to fight ovarian and breast cancers.

Complementary treatments also depend on the wisdom of traditional cultures, from natural immune-boosters like echinacea—the purple cone-flower used by Native Americans—to psychoactive treatments like the antidepressant St. John's Wort (hypericum) from Europe. In the U.S., vast fields of evening primrose are harvested for the gamma-linolenic acid (GLA), thought to stabilize hormonal imbalance, while the fruit of the Asian ginkgo biloba tree gives a fillip to circulation and memory by improving blood flow to the body and brain.

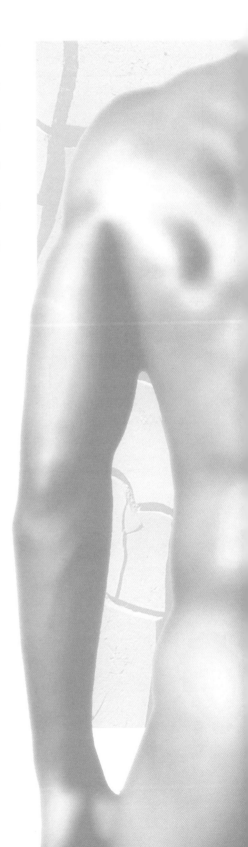

natural healers

Here are some common plants used for their medicinal qualities. Each has its own method of application, and you might want to consult a herbal practitioner before using any of them.

Aloe (*Aloe vera*): A tropical plant, used to heal wounds, as a sedative, and as purgative. It also has tonic and antifungal effects.

Cayenne chili (*Capsicum frutescens*): Used for adding heat to spicy food, the chili stimulates circulation and promotes healing.

Ginger (*Zingiber officinalis*): Popular in cooking, ginger stimulates circulation, counteracts nausea and has an anti-inflammatory action.

earth

grow your own

Most of these herbal medicines are processed into tablets and tinctures, so it is hard to tell natural ingredients from those synthesized in a laboratory. But why not start your own medicinal garden and grow your own crop of natural healers? Many medicinal herbs are sturdy annuals that are easy to grow, even in a pot or window box. They often have attractive foliage or appealing flowers that add color and scent to your home.

Cultivating herbs and vegetables allows you to take advantage of the natural balance of the whole plant, rather than isolated chemicals. Dandelions are a good example: Although they are naturally diuretic, they contain potassium to restore the body's supplies. It is this holistic quality that makes herbalism so valuable. These are rarely quick-fix remedies, so it is often best to incorporate them into your lifestyle if you can. For example, add medicinal plants to your diet, sip herbal teas in place of coffee and use floral rinses to keep skin complaints at bay.

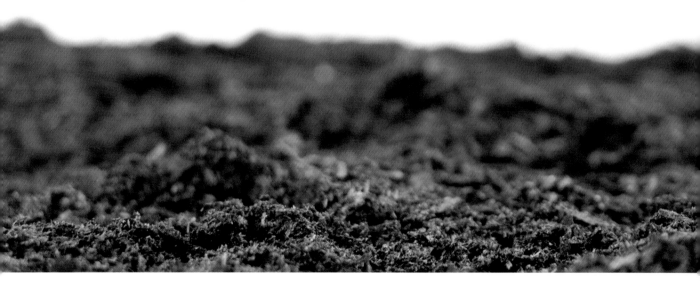

There are a number of different ways that you can apply your herbal medicines. You could prepare an infusion by simply pouring boiling water over the freshly-picked leaves, or a decoction, which involves boiling the plant in water to extract its goodness. Various herbs also lend themselves to tinctures, syrups, oils, cold infusions, creams, ointments, powders, compresses, and poultices. Check how each herb should be applied before using it.

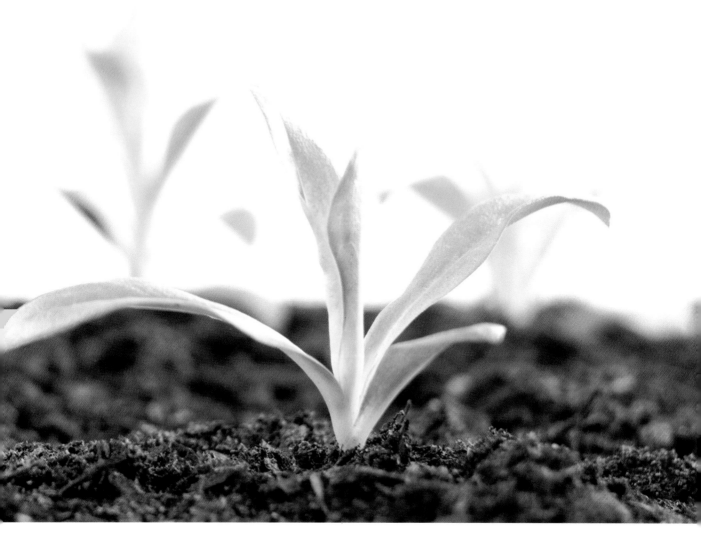

earth

pick your own

To enjoy the benefits of these natural medicines to the full, it is best to harvest them yourself. Most herbs flower in spring and summer, so air dry some at home by hanging them in bunches to use out of season.

Chamomile contains a soothing bioflavonoid that can counter stress and stomach upsets. There are two varieties, both with daisy-like flowers, but the tiny Roman chamomile (*Anthemis nobilis*) is the best: It can

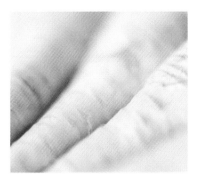

also be used as a fragrant lawn. Infuse ten fresh flowers in a mug of boiled water for ten minutes, then strain and drink. For a delicious summer drink, serve it chilled and mixed with pineapple juice. This mixture is doubly effective for indigestion, thanks to the enzymes the pineapple contains. Combined, they make a totally relaxing and fragrant summer drink.

Peppermint is a traditional cure for indigestion. Spearmint makes a sweet, refreshing tea though black mint is stronger—try several varieties to see which suits you best. Mint is easy to grow and can become invasive, so plant it in a pot or a bucket buried beneath the soil. Pick mint for drying on a sunny summer day before it flowers, and hang it up in small bunches. Rub

the dried leaves between your hands and store in an airtight jar. To make mint tea, add a heaped teaspoon of fresh leaves to a mug of boiled water and leave for ten minutes before drinking.

Pot marigold (calendula) flowers throughout summer and fall, and will seed itself, although it is best to buy fresh seed every year. You can make it into a rinse to comfort sore skin and eczema by steeping four ounces of fresh marigold heads in a pint of freshly boiled water. After it has cooled, strain it and apply with muslin or cotton wool. Red sage grows well with pot marigold. Use the purplish leaves for a gargle to calm a sore throat. Add two heaped teaspoons to a mug of freshly boiled water and infuse for ten minutes before straining.

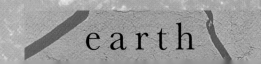

earth

natural first aid

Herbal remedies have been used for years to treat wounds and minor ailments and their popularity in this area is increasing as people discover how effective they can be.

skin

Arnica works wonders for sprains, bruises, and aching joints. Buy it as cream or a tincture (liquid) made from whole plants, but avoid using it on broken skin. Comfrey is available as a cream or root that can be used as a poultice to heal sores. Neither arnica nor comfrey should ever be taken internally, unlike goldenseal, which is excellent for both wounds and sore throats. A cut aloe vera leaf or gel will soothe burns, including sunburn, and raw honey has been found to speed healing in both burns and wounds. Vitamin E rubbed into the skin is another way to heal cuts and also prevents scarring. Use natural vitamin E (d-alpha-tocopherol).

If skin irritation is the problem, try calendula (marigold) cream on sore, flaking skin, including eczema. For skin infections, one of the most versatile remedies is Australian tea tree oil. Its antibacterial, antifungal action makes it ideal for inflammation, spots and athlete's foot. Essential oil of lavender also helps fight infection—use it neat on spots and insect bites. You can also turn to the antibacterial powers of garlic and cabbage to beat skin infections such as acne. (Test for sensitivity using your elbow.) To prepare the cabbage, liquefy eight ounces of fresh leaves, strain and add two drops of lemon oil. Use this mixture as a lotion applied directly to the affected area, allowing the lotion to sit for a few moments before rinsing it off. For the garlic, simply rub the affected area with a cut clove.

digestion

Slippery elm, marshmallow, and licorice soothe the membranes and help repair the lining of the gut, so take them after a bout of food poisoning. Gentian (bitters) is an excellent aid to digestion, which is why cocktails made with angostura bitters, Campari, gin and bitter lemon are traditional aperitifs. If nausea is a problem, one of the most effective remedies is ginger. Make a tea from grated root ginger or chew crystallized ginger for travel sickness.

insomnia

Hops are the traditional cure for insomnia and they can be taken as capsules or used in a pillow if you do not like beer. Lettuce can be used for its soporific effects too, but the most powerful natural sedative is the herb valerian. Although you can buy the root, it is best taken as capsules or tincture in order to regulate the dose. Valerian is a potent medicine and should be taken in strictly controlled quantities.

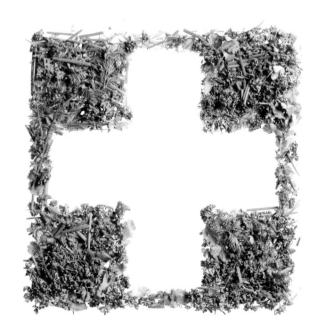

earth

plant warriors

Concern about the overuse of antibiotics is at last putting an end to their use for mild respiratory disease and sore throats, which in any case are often viral and will not respond to these drugs. Antibiotics have proved weaker than the bacteria they aim to kill and their routine use in both animals and humans has been blamed for the growth of "superbugs"—resistant staphylococcus infections such as MRSA, too often a life-threatening consequence of hospital treatment. However, while you may agree that antibiotics are overprescribed, it is a different matter when you are suffering with an inflamed throat or a cold that won't go away. Luckily there is a whole arsenal of powerful natural remedies that can come to the rescue.

first

A number of remedies can work when symptoms first strike. They include echinacea, which, taken at the first tickle of a cold can stop infection in its tracks. (Remember: Do not take it "just in case," as it becomes ineffective with prolonged use.) Garlic is a powerful antibacterial, best eaten raw. Newer to the West are the Chinese herb astralgus and the African potato, which maintains the number of disease-fighting white blood cells in the body.

next

Infection is more difficult to shift once it is established but natural methods can help. For infections of the throat and digestive tract, try citricidal or extract of grapefruit seeds, which has an immensely powerful antioxidant action. Some remedies have a very specific action: Cranberries, for example, are used to treat cystitis because the berries contain an acid that stops bacteria clinging to the bladder walls.

for the future

Building up resistance to infection is one of the best ways to fight off

infection. You can protect yourself with foods rich

in antioxidant vitamins and zinc but

another way to build up your

immunity is by taking Siberian

ginseng (*eleutherococcus*) not

to be confused with stimulant

ginseng or panax, which has long-term

benefits for health.

earth

scents of well-being

Open a tiny bottle of essential oil, shake a few drops into oil or water, and inhale the fragrance of a field full of flowers. This is aromatherapy, the centuries-old art of healing with essential oils. Over two hundred plants, from blossoms and flowers to herbs and roots, yield up their perfume and each has a different value—in more ways than one. Though some plants, such as frankincense and lavender, have a plentiful supply of oil, it can take thousands of rose petals or millions of jasmine flowers to create just a few ounces of their precious and highly scented essence.

Soaking in a scented bath or giving yourself up to a rhythmic aromatherapy massage must be the most indulgent ways to treat both mind and body. This is why aromatherapy is practiced in so many centers dedicated to well-being, from health spas and beauty clinics to holistic medical centers and hospices. Because the sense of smell links to the limbic system in the brain, which controls mood, and is close to the memory centers, aromatherapy has the power to unlock the emotions. Along with euphoria and joy can come a welcome bout of tears.

Although every oil is unique, their qualities overlap and two or three can be blended to create a healing aromatic cocktail. If you feel tense, irritable or upset, choose from clary, lavender, neroli, rose, or ylang-ylang, all of which can help you relax. If you are exhausted and drained of energy both mentally and physically, pick basil, orange, and rosemary to revive yourself. And if you want to choose a single oil to explore this fascinating therapy, try geranium, which has the power to calm and rebalance the system.

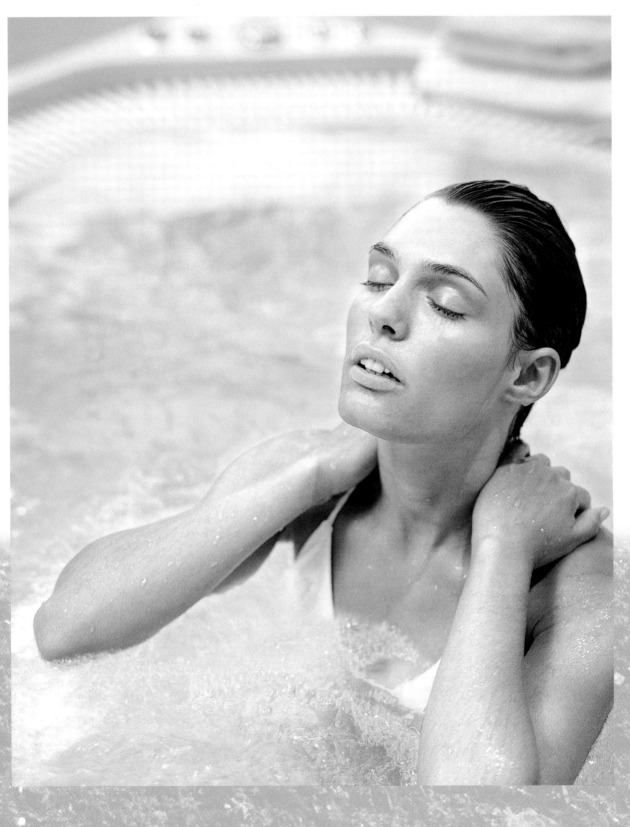

earth

to hug and to hold

When words are not enough, we resort to touch. Clasped hands, a kiss, and an embrace are not only for lovers. They

reassure us that we are cared for and that we are not alone, which is why a fleeting touch on the elbow is enough to make

us feel warmer toward the toucher.

This is the philosophy that supports massage and the therapies that rely on touch. Along with practical skills like

unknotting tight muscles and realigning bones, the best practitioners transmit a healing power through their hands.

Their gifts are confirmed by research, which concludes that massage can reduce anxiety and tension, help wounds

heal faster, promote lymph drainage after breast cancer, and even, according to the University of Miami's Touch

Research Institute, encourage premature babies to thrive.

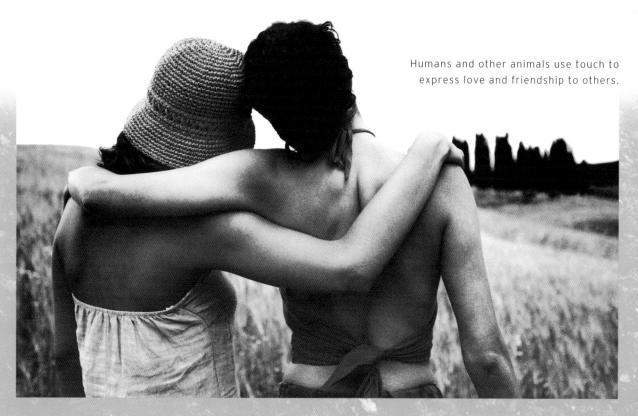

Humans and other animals use touch to
express love and friendship to others.

Originally, the main aims of massage were to improve blood flow and ease stiff joints. But although physical release and pain relief are still the aims of traditional Swedish massage, osteopathy, and chiropractic, recently there has been a move away from simple manipulation to methods where subtle degrees of touch are used to restore the body and refresh the soul.

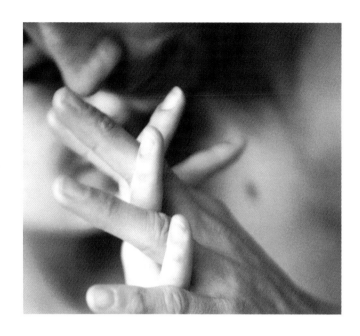

Some, such as spiritual healing or therapeutic touch, depend completely on the transference of healing energy, with or without the laying on of hands. Others, such as shiatsu and Reiki, aim to access the life-force or "chi" in the body by applying pressure to specific points. There are an increasing number of new therapies in which ideas from traditional bodywork are filtered and adapted: Examples are the Bowen technique (a rolling, rebalancing massage), McTimoney (a gentle take on chiropractic) and Feldenkrais, which reworks movements. Although you should explore them as much as you wish, because bodywork has the power to harm as well as heal, always check the qualifications and experience of therapists before committing yourself to treatment with them. Ask how they would help your particular problem, whether their approach is purely physical or designed to encourage emotional release, and if you will be clothed or naked. A sense of trust in the therapist is essential.

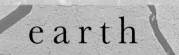

earth

the fragrant touch

Just as a professional aromatherapist will assess the state of your mind and body before treating you, so can you

learn to tune in to your feelings and correct imbalances with essential oils. Work with a partner or friend if you can,

to benefit from another's touch. Atmosphere is important, so put on some soothing new age music, birdsong, or a

gentle classic like *Gymnopedies* (Erik Satie) or *Walk to the Paradise Garden* (Frederick Delius). Pile up the fluffiest

towels you can find to cover yourself and the couch, and make sure that the room, and your hands, are comfortably

warm so that you can be both naked and relaxed.

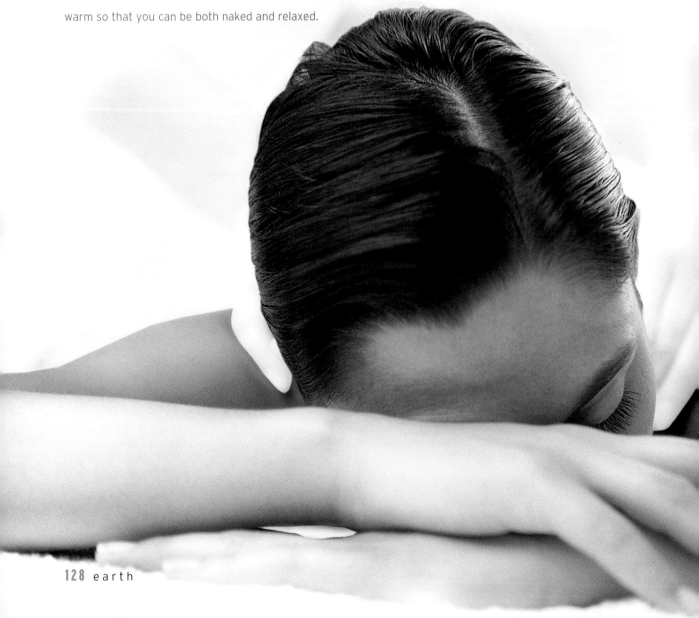

aromatherapy *à deux*

For a massage guaranteed to leave you feeling languorous and trouble-free, blend four teaspoons of warmed sweet almond oil with three drops of antidepressant essential oil of rose, three of rebalancing geranium, and three of anxiety-relieving neroli—orange blossom. Because essential oils are so powerful, they are always mixed with a neutral carrier oil, which provides lubrication and prevents irritation, allowing the fragrance to seep slowly into the skin.

Treat your partner with this soothing massage. Rub the oil between your palms, and using the whole of your hand, press either side of the spine with long firm strokes, moving up toward the neck and down each side. Avoid putting pressure on the spine, throat, or any broken veins. Work along the limbs in the direction of the heart with smooth strokes, except when pulling gently on the fingers and toes. When the muscles are warm, graduate to kneading movements but use only the lightest touch on the face and belly, which can be stroked in a gentle clockwise movement. Now gradually relax the pressure with slower strokes, finishing with featherlight caresses. Now it is your turn... and at the end of the massage, cover yourself with a warm towel and relax deeply, or allow yourself to drift off to sleep.

no partner?

You can treat yourself—drizzle a little oil down your back and use a long-handled wooden roller to massage each side of your spine.

earth

head to toe

Concentrating on a single part of the body can improve the health of the whole. Take cranial osteopathy and craniosacral therapy, where subtle pressure is applied to the head. These treatments are so gentle that in the hands of a skilled therapist you can hardly feel the shifts that take place inside the skull. Even so, advocates say it can relieve headache and pain after injury, and help young children overcome problems caused by birth trauma. One of the oldest therapies, the Alexander Technique, concentrates on spinal alignment to restore upright posture, deep breathing, and good health. The rewards include a reduction in stress-related illness such as headache, backache, indigestion, and depression.

cranial osteopathy

This gentle therapy works on the subtle manipulation of the cranium. The theory is that the skull suffers considerable trauma at birth, which can lead to chronic problems later on in life. The manipulation of the skull aims to release pressure in the brain.

alexander technique

Developed in the nineteenth century by Frederick Alexander, the Alexander Technique aims to help people recover more natural posture and movement. It focuses particularly on achieving a proper alignment of the spine. The technique has been adopted by many other therapies.

reflexology

Based on the ancient Chinese system of medicine, reflexology works on the principle that the energy lines that run through the body are represented in the feet and the hands. Practitioners manipulate the palms of the hands and the soles of the feet to diagnose and treat physical problems.

Bodywork can also be diagnostic. In reflexology, which is based on the Chinese medicinal understanding of the body, the feet and hands act as a mirror of the body, and tenderness in a particular area can point to problems in the organs. Similarly, kinesiology tests muscle strength, health, and flexibility to check for problems that exist elsewhere in the body.

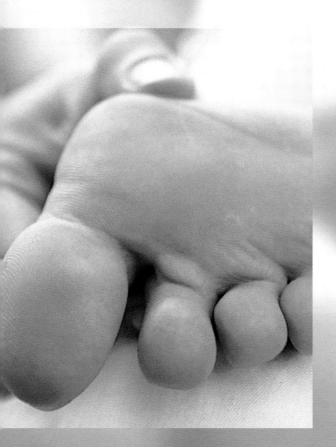

kinesiology

This therapy focuses on feedback from the muscles to diagnose and treat physical and mental problems. The goal of kinesiology is to achieve a balanced whole between the various parts of the body and the various parts of the mind. Numerous forms of kinesiology are practiced today.

earth

simple self-massage

Here is a simple routine to relieve tension and stiffness in the upper body.

Shrug your shoulders toward your ears and release, then put

your hands on your shoulders and circle your elbows forward

and back to gently massage your shoulders.

Clasp your right arm with your left hand above the elbow,

thumb upward. Press into the muscle and work gently

upward, then move your hand under your arm and work your

thumb into the muscle just below the shoulder, moving from

side to side. Cross your right arm in front of you and squeeze

the back of your upper arm with your left hand, moving

toward the elbow. Repeat on the other side.

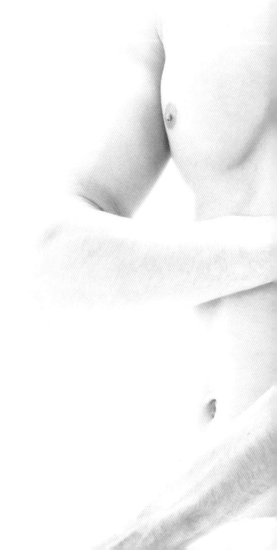

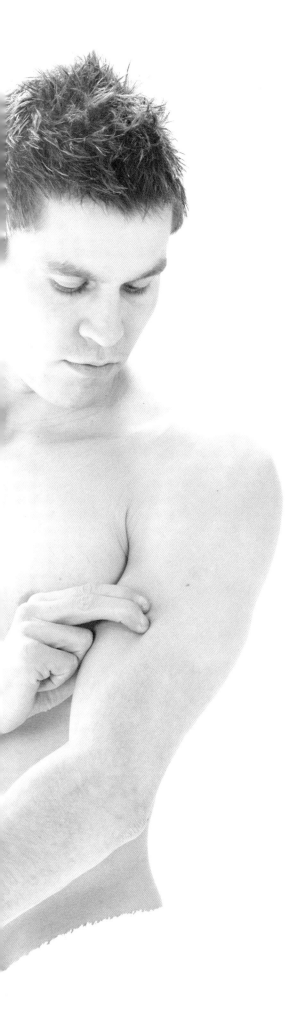

Put your hands in your lap and breathe deeply. Stretch out your neck, then alternately raise and dip your chin, returning to the center each time. Cross your left arm over your chest and massage the muscle below the base of your skull. Drag your hand along the shoulder as you tilt your head the opposite way. Repeat on the other side. Tug your ear lobes and gently pinch round the rim of your ear. Rub your hands briskly and place them over your eyes. Pinch gently along your eyebrows between the thumb and forefinger.

Pat your head with floppy fingers, working from front to back. Finish by sweeping your palms over your head and shoulders.

earth

fire

Fire destroys but it also creates. Fire gives
us light, and without the warmth of the sun,
the earth would be a frozen planet incapable
of sustaining life. Fire also exists deep within
the earth, whose molten core has the power
to reshape continents. And while fire lays
waste, it also purifies, making way for new
life and new beginnings.

rebirth
Like electricity, thoughts crackle between the nerve cells in the brain, providing the creative **impulse** that produces art, music, literature, and philosophy. It is this **fire** within that expresses who we are, and which needs constant refuelling if it is to burn brightly.

fire

release your creativity

It may flicker, but there is a creative flame inside everyone. Simply humming a tune, cooking a dish, or sending an e-mail gives shape to your thoughts, which is the essence of creativity. However, the creative impulse is fragile and easily crushed. A discouraging response to a child's painting (What's it supposed to be?) can put an end to her exuberant play with colors, patterns, and shapes, while a flunked music or dancing exam may be enough to instill a permanent sense of failure. However, despite these negative experiences, it is possible to repair the damaging effects of criticism.

fire

open your mind

Flexible thinking is essential for a creative breakthrough. Brainstorming, where every idea is valued and nothing condemned as trivial, is a kind of flexible thinking. Practice by creating an ideas file, where you note down any ideas that come into your head and see how you can use them to shape your thinking, and maybe your life. Above all, communicate. Speak to people who differ in age and culture from yourself whenever you have the opportunity—it will enrich your mind with ideas outside your own experience. Receiving ideas should be an active process. Limit TV and Internet surfing to a maximum of 90 minutes a day, and increase the time you spend reading.

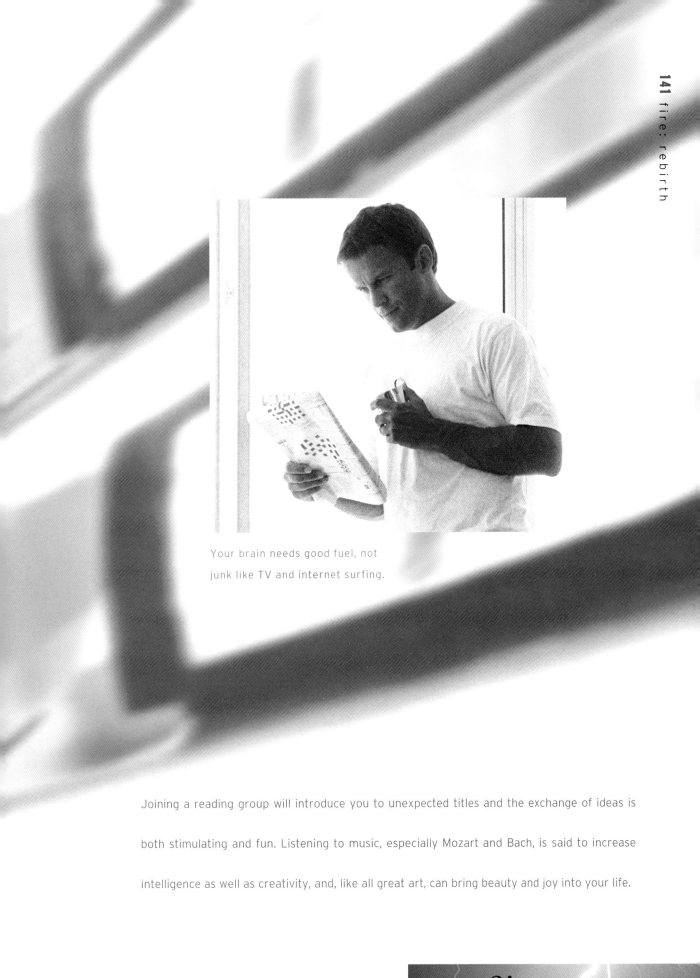

Your brain needs good fuel, not junk like TV and internet surfing.

Joining a reading group will introduce you to unexpected titles and the exchange of ideas is both stimulating and fun. Listening to music, especially Mozart and Bach, is said to increase intelligence as well as creativity, and, like all great art, can bring beauty and joy into your life.

fire

the secret of play

Young creatures, from kittens to children, learn through play. As they frolic about, they learn to relate to each other, absorb information, and imitate the adult world, practicing skills they will need later in life.

So, time to act like a child again. New experiences stick in the memory, so seek out something new every day—a new taste, a new street, a new way of doing things. A change of perspective challenges the imagination and can stimulate your creativity. Try some simple transformation tricks by making an ikebana arrangement from stones and twigs, folding paper into origami shapes, or painting a piece of furniture with your own design.

Pretending is one part of play that persists in adult life, but too often it is a cover for insecurity. Confidence games like "My Hero" provide a positive spin. Imagine you are someone you admire and next time you are assailed by doubts, behave as you think they would.

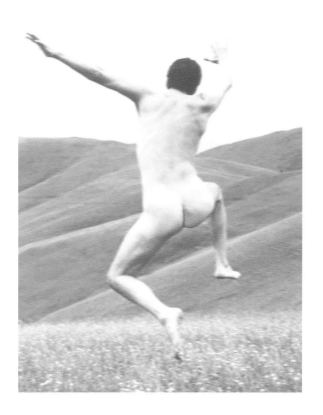

act on impulse

Weighing up the pros and cons and arriving at a balanced judgment is a mature skill, which is why forgetting it can be such a buzz. You don't have to go bungee jumping or do extreme sports. Try running until you are out of breath, splashing in a stream or in the sea, or swinging idly from a branch—anything that is pointless, harmless, and completely unproductive. Indulging your instincts helps strip away the conditioning that wraps round you like an invisible veil, setting your thoughts free.

fire

sparking ideas

Just as exercise tones the body, so mind games can improve the brain. They provide a quick route to creativity when thought processes seem blocked and keep the mind sharp and agile: Research shows that having an absorbing interest, especially if you're over 40, protects against memory loss and mental decay. Far from being a process that is complete soon after birth, new neural connections are developed throughout life. With learning, practice, and flexibility, you really can reshape your brain.

Many mind games aim to extend the brain's capacity by creating new links. Routine can make your mind rigid; if you always drive to work the same way, the road becomes so familiar that it is easy to journey for miles without noticing the landmarks. Varying the routes your thinking takes builds new mental maps and helps improve spatial skills.

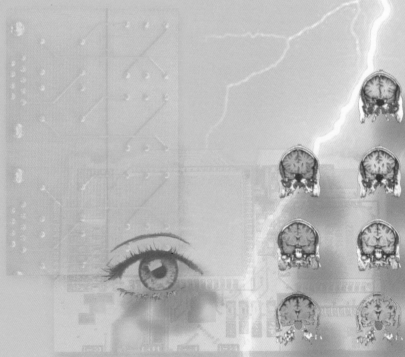

Neural cross-training is another way to break established patterns. This exercises the brain cells on your non-dominant side. If you are right-handed, try eating and dressing with your left, and vice versa. Sketch an object with your dominant hand and then try with your other hand. Now compare them—and prepare to be spooked. Or take up dancing—for example, Scottish dancing, ballet, or salsa. Crossing your feet and then trying to change direction will invigorate both brain and body.

Learning a language stimulates the brain cells, but so does a word workout in your own language. Reading silently, listening to words, and reading aloud exercise different parts of the brain. While silent reading uses just one area in the left side of the brain, listening to words activates both hemispheres, and reading aloud involves the areas needed for physical coordination.

fire

creative thinking

A trained mind is a contradiction in terms; to be creative, we need to think beyond the conventional, questioning not only what we learn but also the way we learn it. In the West, logical thought and linear progression—properties of the analytical left side of the brain—are emphasized and valued the most. Sometimes we need to disengage this side of the brain in favor of the creative and free-ranging right.

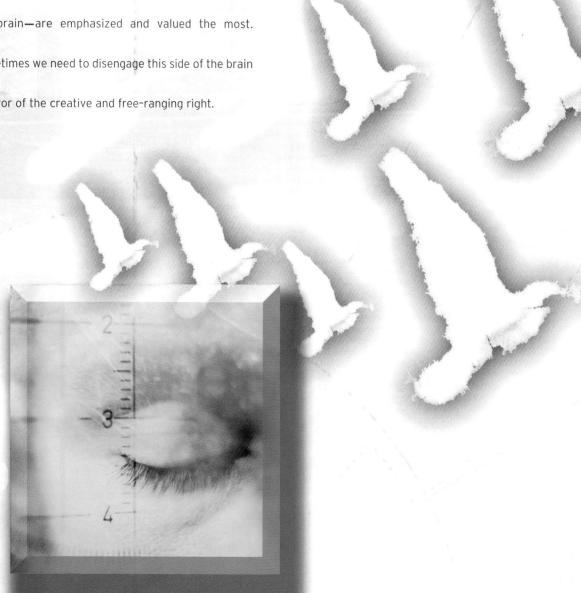

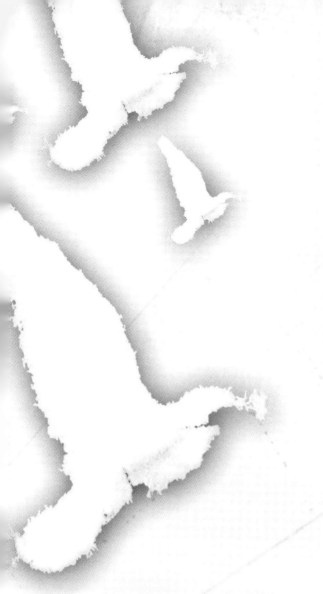

To tap into our creative abilities we need to unlearn many ways in which we have grown accustomed to thinking and viewing ourselves and the world.

It was the geography of the brain that prompted the idea of mind-mapping, or thought association, as an aid to learning. A page or screen has a format that is quite different from the intricate network of neurons inside the brain, and mirroring these can release creativity, the theory goes. Instead of making notes in a structured way, simply write down a central idea and work in all directions, setting down thoughts in clusters that spiral outward from the core. Although it sounds chaotic, it can promote creative thinking and help reveal the whole picture rather than just a part.

Setting free the creative part of the brain can also allay anxiety, because visualization is an important aid to relaxation. Thinking of a peaceful scene—a secluded beach on a sunny day, say—distracts the mind from worrying or obsessive thoughts. Concentrating on each element—imagining the trickle of sand beneath the feet, the warmth of the breeze and the sound of birds calling—can help release tension, lower heart rate, and instill a deep sense of calm.

fire

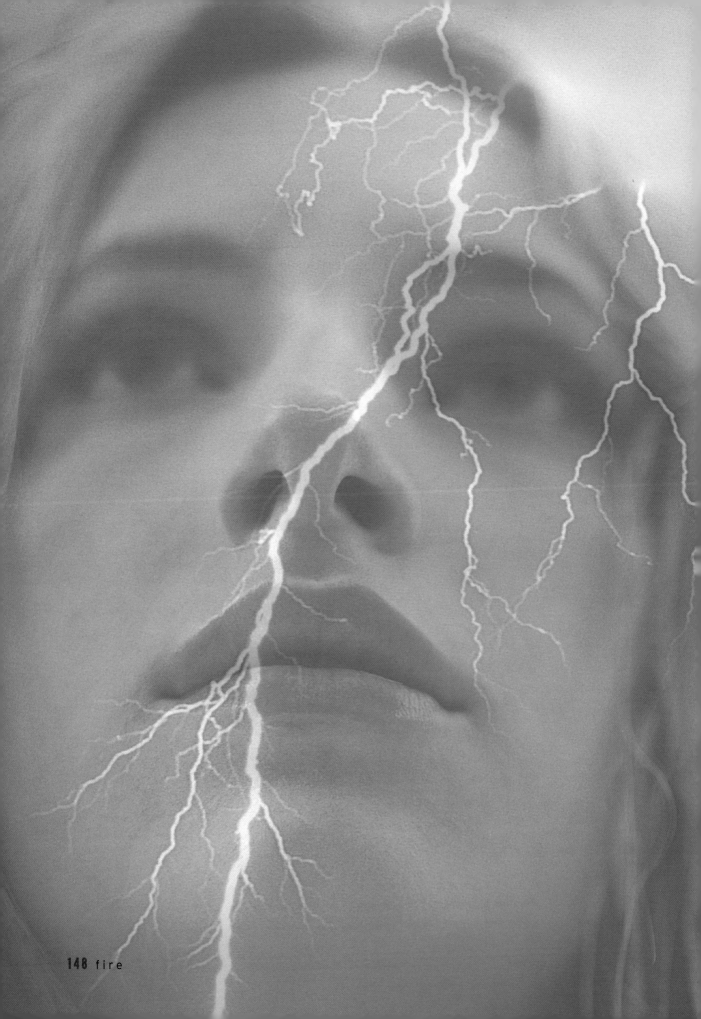

energy Lightning rips through the sky, thunder peals, and the temperature and atmospheric pressure tumble—the **energy** released by a **storm** is almost palpable, and can have consequences for both mind and body. We need to be able to access the dynamic energy within us.

fire

revitalize yourself

healing nights

One woman in three complains of constant fatigue, a condition known as TATT—Tired All The Time. And what is behind this modern epidemic? There is nothing mysterious about "unexplained" fatigue; too little sleep, relaxation, and exercise coupled with too much work, worry, and stress is the classic recipe for burnout. To recharge, take a break from routine. Book a short trip away, and then another. Schedule in about six breaks a year—a weekend will do—varying the type and destination of each vacation.

While American physicians call for a Bill of Nights in which everyone has eight hours of sleep a night, the reality is that many people make do with six hours. For some, that may be enough, but if you have to be roused by an alarm and wake up exhausted, consider this. Lack of sleep increases cortisol, the stress hormone. It can deplete the

nothing doing

immune system, increasing susceptibility to colds and flu, accelerate age-related conditions like diabetes and high blood pressure, and plays havoc with memory and thinking. All the more reason, then, to treat yourself to sufficient sleep.

In a twilight state of deep relaxation, the brain's rhythms change; it is at this time that we are most likely to experience a "eureka" breakthrough. Find time for some deep relaxation. Take at least half an hour every day to indulge your senses—try soaking in a scented bath, people-watching in the park or listening to music with 60 beats a minute to slow the brainwaves to a rate similar to meditation.

fire

raw energy

Food is fuel for the body, and calories are the units of energy in which it is measured. However, that does not mean that high-cal foods are the best choice for boosting energy—in fact, the reverse can be true. A heavy meal packed with lots of calories that diverts blood from the brain can induce drowsiness, and though a quick sugar-fix chocolate bar is tempting when hunger strikes and will provide a quick energy boost, the rebound effect can make you feel faint and jittery. There are kinder ways to help your mind feel alert and your body full of energy.

slow-release ten slow-release energy foods

1 brown rice

2 oats

3 potatoes

4 broccoli

5 cauliflower

6 apples/pears

7 wholegrain bread

8 sprouts

9 mushrooms

10 berries

hard day ahead?

For lasting stamina, you need the slow-release energy provided by complex carbohydrates like wholegrain cereals, potatoes, brown rice, pasta, and wholegrain bread. The gradual process of converting these into sugar during digestion keeps glucose levels steady and prevents energy fluctuation. And you really do need breakfast: Research shows that concentration and thinking flag without it. So start the day with sugar-free muesli, porridge, or thick slices of wholegrain toast and fresh fruit, to power both body and brain.

quick-fix ten healthy quick-fix energy foods

1 tomatoes

2 figs

3 bananas

4 oranges

5 dried fruit

6 nuts

7 grapes

8 prunes

9 raw peppers

10 raw carrots

fire

natural stimulants

There are several herbs that can give your system a boost. At times when you feel

low as well as shattered, eat basil, known for its uplifting quality. A course

of ginseng (panax) may make you feel more resilient but it is not a quick fix.

Although it's a well-known tonic and sexual stimulant, it does need to be taken for

several months.

Because magnesium helps release energy and plays a role in controlling

temperature, nerves, and muscles, it is wise to increase your intake by eating

more wholegrains, nuts, and seeds. And if you are still exhausted, ask your doctor

to check your hemoglobin count to see if iron supplements, or regular servings of

liver, are necessary to stave off anemia.

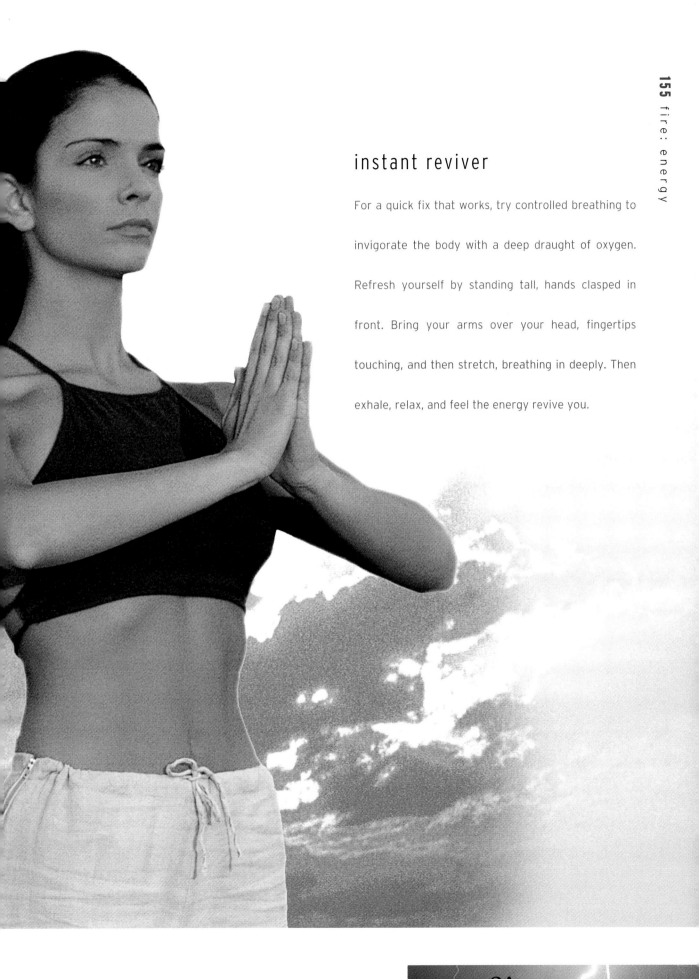

instant reviver

For a quick fix that works, try controlled breathing to

invigorate the body with a deep draught of oxygen.

Refresh yourself by standing tall, hands clasped in

front. Bring your arms over your head, fingertips

touching, and then stretch, breathing in deeply. Then

exhale, relax, and feel the energy revive you.

fire

burning energy

Exercise is a fast, free way to have a total makeover. Your skin glows, thanks to the surge of oxygen-rich blood pumped out by the heart, and fat is converted into energy as the metabolism speeds up (and remains higher even after exercise is over). Muscles become better defined and bone loss is slowed, improving shape and posture. As the oxygen-laden blood reaches your brain, the mind clears and endorphins are released, creating a feeling of euphoria.

nice 'n' easy

Although most benefits are usually associated with aerobic exercise, which raises the heart rate and gets you sweating, new findings show that leisurely exercise is valuable too. The total amount of time spent active is more important than its intensity, according to a study of 40,000 women by Harvard Medical School, which found that

calories burned

15 minutes		30 minutes	
aerobics	105 calories	aerobics	215 calories
jogging	125 calories	jogging	250 calories
running uphill or upstairs	270 calories	running uphill or upstairs	535 calories
gardening	90 calories	gardening	180 calories
swimming	145 calories	swimming	285 calories
brisk walking	80 calories	brisk walking	160 calories

the risk of heart disease can be halved by walking for an hour a week. Any exercise can get the circulation working at an increased rate and so improve the health of the heart. Exercise is valuable at any age, because it keeps the mind lively throughout life. Just half an hour's moderate activity a day burns as much as 1000 calories a week.

move your body

To get full enjoyment from your food, it is important to revel in the energy it creates. Exercise has become a leisure activity and every year sees a new craze, from line dancing to tae kwan do. If you like change, company, and motivation, one of these could be right for you. If you prefer to go at your own pace, combine walking or cycling with exploring a new region or even a new country, challenging the mind as well as the body.

45 minutes

aerobics	**320 calories**
jogging	**375 calories**
running uphill or upstairs	**805 calories**
gardening	**270 calories**
swimming	**430 calories**
brisk walking	**240 calories**

60 minutes

aerobics	**429 calories**
jogging	**501 calories**
running uphill or upstairs	**1074 calories**
gardening	**358 calories**
swimming	**572 calories**
brisk walking	**322 calories**

fire

the naked shape

Exercise not only feels good, it helps you to look good too—sculpting the body to peel flab from thighs and arms, flattening the belly, and lifting the butt. The most marked effects come from a combination of aerobic exercise, which burns fat, with strength training to tone muscles and stretching for flexibility. To decide which exercise system is best for you, pinch a little slack flesh—on your upper arm, say—between your fingers, then flex the muscle behind. If your skin becomes smooth and taut, think about using weights to build up muscle. If you're holding a handful of fat, concentrate on aerobic exercise. An hourly session four times a week will help you shape up fast, but half that amount will also have a noticeable impact in time. The trick is to be consistent.

It is worth seeking out a good, soft, but supportive surface to run on. Running on concrete is to be avoided, as it jars the body and increases the wear on joints.

fast track workouts

Running is free, it gets you out in the fresh air, and it is one of the quickest ways to improve your shape and fitness. Pounding the streets is hard on the joints, so cushion your feet and knees by swapping the road for grass or a dirt track, which provide a softer landing, and alternate running with walking to lower the impact on your limbs. Though running barefoot in the park or the beach is fine occasionally, always wear supportive shoes for serious running.

If you prefer a class but are sick of step aerobics, consider taking up kick boxing. Ideal for channeling aggression and getting rid of stress, this powerful whole-body workout combines classic boxing (gloves, pads, feinting, and parrying) with martial arts kicks. For non-contact sport, try ashtanga (power yoga), which introduces speed and energy to classic yoga sequences. And if you want to avoid traffic fumes, consider spinning—synchronized exercise bikes.

learn to love it

A creative approach to exercise can increase your enjoyment. You don't have to go to a gym to experience karaoke cycling or disco yoga. Try them at home, and make up your own variants. Anyone for disco tennis?

fire

inner strength

There is a method of exercise that defines your shape yet won't make you sweat, puff, or strain your back. Pilates,

named after the man who developed the technique, has become one of the most popular forms of body conditioning.

It relies on controlled movements so slight as to be almost imperceptible, but don't be fooled. The movements are

designed to work the deep muscles, so it is more forceful than it looks. Correct breathing

and alignment are vital parts of this technique and must be mastered before any

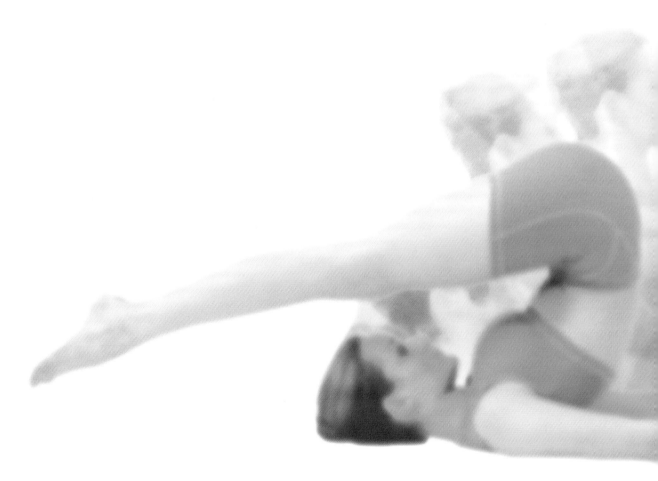

exercise can start; disciples soon become familiar with requests to check that their feet are parallel and to pull 'navel to spine'. Are there any drawbacks? Well it can be slow, so if you like a fast or vigorous workout it is probably not for you. And because special equipment is needed for the full range of movements, the class may be restricted and less interesting if this is not available. Otherwise, it is an ideal way to improve strength and flexibility, leaving you physically tired but mentally refreshed.

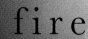
fire

a change of pace

The body is quick to adapt to new demands, so vary the exercises for maximum benefit. A change of style also helps retain your interest and gives your mind a different focus. Dancing (ballet, folk, salsa, ballroom, line—it is up to you), exercise classes, and sports like tennis or golf are more social, while walking or cycling alone offer the chance to think and observe. And if you want time out, try swimming, which can induce a trance-like state similar to meditation.

listen to your heartbeat

To gain from aerobic exercise, you need to get your heart going at between

60 and 95 percent of your normal working range. Use the following

formulas to find your maximum heart rate: for women 209 - (0.9 x age); for

men 214 - (0.8 x age). So a woman who is thirty-two years old would have

a maximum of 180 beats per minute. A man the same age would have 188.

the hostile flame

Energy can be destructive as well as creative. Whether expressed through storms, volcanic eruptions, or human hostility, the results can be devastating. Although there is little you can do to control the forces of nature, anger, at least, can be managed.

Anger is not always a negative emotion. It can also be an agent for good, providing the impetus to put right society's wrongs. But it needs to be channeled—if it is suppressed, it can have a damaging effect on both physical and mental health and there is a risk it will be expressed anyway.

type A person

These Type A personality characteristics describe the classic stressed-out executive. But it can apply to anyone, not just a suit:

commitment to having rather than being

unawareness of things outside their sphere of interest

need to be an expert in a subject, otherwise not interested

sense of being in a hurry all the time

feeling of guilt when relaxing

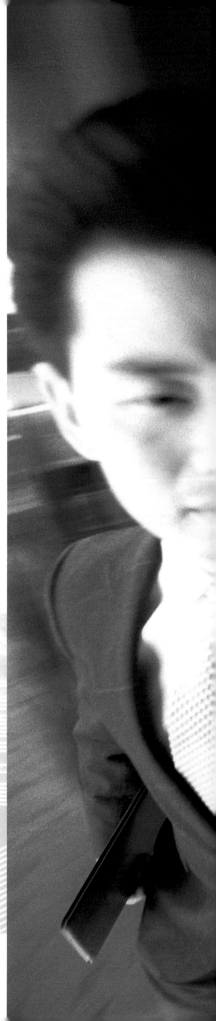

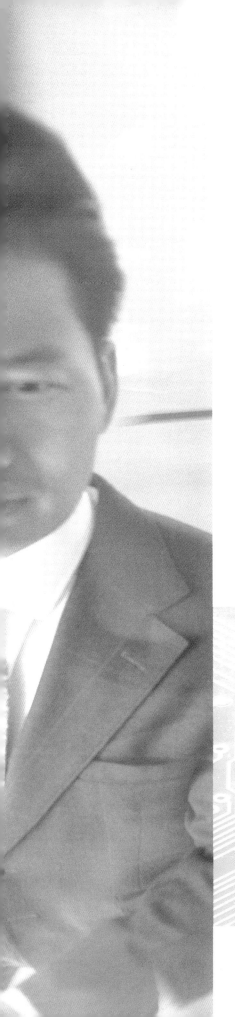

Impatience and hostility have been implicated in causes of high blood pressure and heart disease, something to bear in mind next time you find yourself cursing the driver in front. This classic Type A behavior is a reaction to stress that is becoming more prevalent in the industrialized world's pressured, 24-hour society. Once only associated with high-powered businessmen, Type As are now just as likely to be found in middle management and stressed-out working moms. Why? Long-term studies have shown a link between the high incidence of heart disease among government employees and a sense of powerlessness in their working lives.

type B person

These Type B personality characteristics describe people who are at peace with themselves and don't need external fixes:

commitment to being rather than having

broad awareness

interested in new ideas and subjects

patient

enjoys peace and can relax effectively

be assertive

It has long been known that suppressed anger can lead to depression. Interestingly, low levels of the brain chemical

serotonin are linked to hostility as well as low mood, so it could be an idea to try foods rich in tryptophan (milk and

poultry, say) and carbohydrates, which increase tryptophan levels in the brain, plus the natural antidepressant, St.

John's Wort. However, the key to improved health is to consciously change behavior by transforming passivity or

aggression into assertiveness. This means having the confidence to state your needs and

expect them to be considered. It means remembering that you have the right to say no,

to set your own priorities, hold your own beliefs, and express your feelings; it also means

taking responsibility for your actions and acknowledging your mistakes. Putting your point of view

across in a relaxed, cooperative way defuses stress and reduces resentment, creating a more pleasant

and effective atmosphere all round.

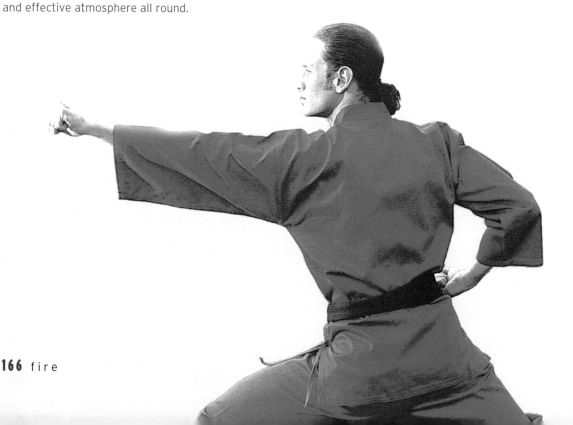

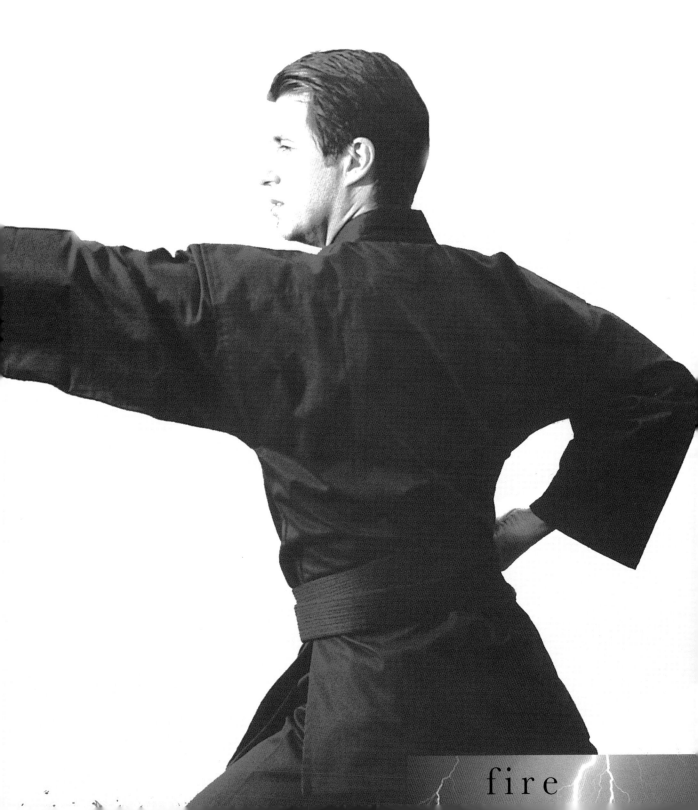

fire

energy medicine

Enlisting the help of natural energy is at the heart of many healing therapies. Sometimes elements outside the body are used to speed up healing, while at other times, a therapy aims to tap into the energy, or life force, inside the body itself.

Energy medicines include homeopathy and Bach flower remedies, which dilute the essence of a chemical or plant so that what remains is little more than an imprint on water. This vibration is thought to convey a healing power, and advocates argue that water can store information in the same way as magnetic media. Sounds fanciful? The jury is still out but experiments have shown that dilute poisons, like those used in homeopathy, can increase animal growth, and that homeopathy is two to three times more powerful than a placebo (dummy pills).

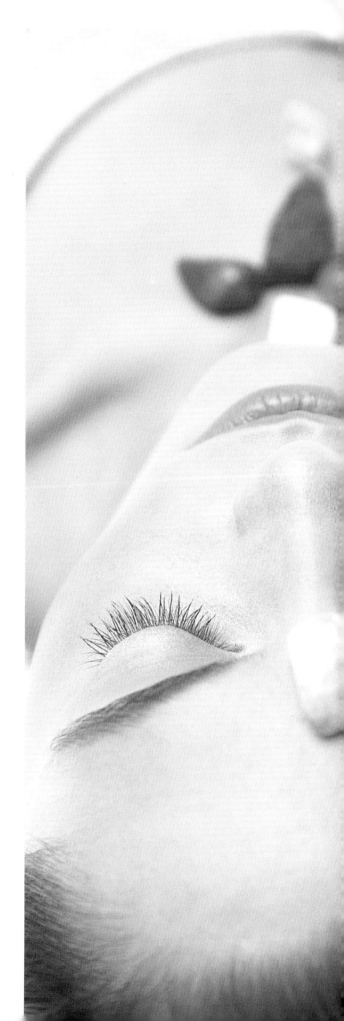

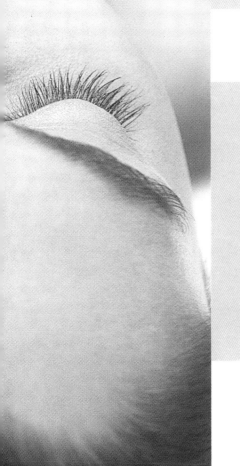

homeopathy

This has many fans, including the British royal family, who are known to take homeopathic medicines on their travels. The theory is that fire drives out fire, so remedies are prescribed which, at full strength, could cause the symptoms being treated. Although you can use homeopathy simply to treat the symptoms of illness, personality plays an important role. Aconite, for example, is best suited to anxious people. This holistic approach, along with the time the homeopath spends analyzing problems, contributes to the therapy's success.

Bach flower remedies

Designed to treat negative feelings (all 38 of them) and the symptoms that these negative feelings cause. Choose clematis if you cannot concentrate, busy lizzy for impatience, centaury if you're anxious to please. Several flower essences can be taken at the same time to suit your mood, and there is also a compound Rescue Remedy, which is taken at times of crisis to restore equilibrium.

fire

attraction of opposites

Electromagnetic energy is a force to be reckoned with. On a global scale, it is responsible for the earth's magnetic field. Locally, it can create mayhem during geomagnetic storms in which the earth is bombarded by high-energy particles from the sun. It is also present at a microscopic level within the body's cells.

It is this internal magnetism that inspires magnetic therapy. Some scientists believe that by applying magnets to an injury, red blood corpuscles are attracted to the area, encouraging healing by improving the oxygen supply and removing harmful wastes. Strong pulses of electromagnetic energy are regularly used to repair fractures and treat deep wounds, and studies are taking place to see if electromagnetism (not to be confused with electro-convulsive, or electric shock, therapy) can relieve migraine and depression. Magnetism is also an important diagnostic tool—magnetic resonance imaging (MRI) produces a sharp picture of the body's bones and organs without any of the hazards of radiation. Research is also underway to find the extent of the electromagnetic system in the body.

So can you be certain that magnetic plasters will soothe pain or a magnetic pillow will help you sleep? Sadly no, because the magnetic stimulation used in hospitals is far stronger than that provided by an ordinary magnet, as anyone who has been surprised by the tremendous clashing and banging during an MRI scan will know. But there is evidence that such devices may help, because research on magnetic insoles shows that in diabetics they help relieve foot pain, a sign of impaired circulation. If you want a natural, painless way to heal that relies on the body's own resources to act as its treatment, magnetic therapy could well be worth a try.

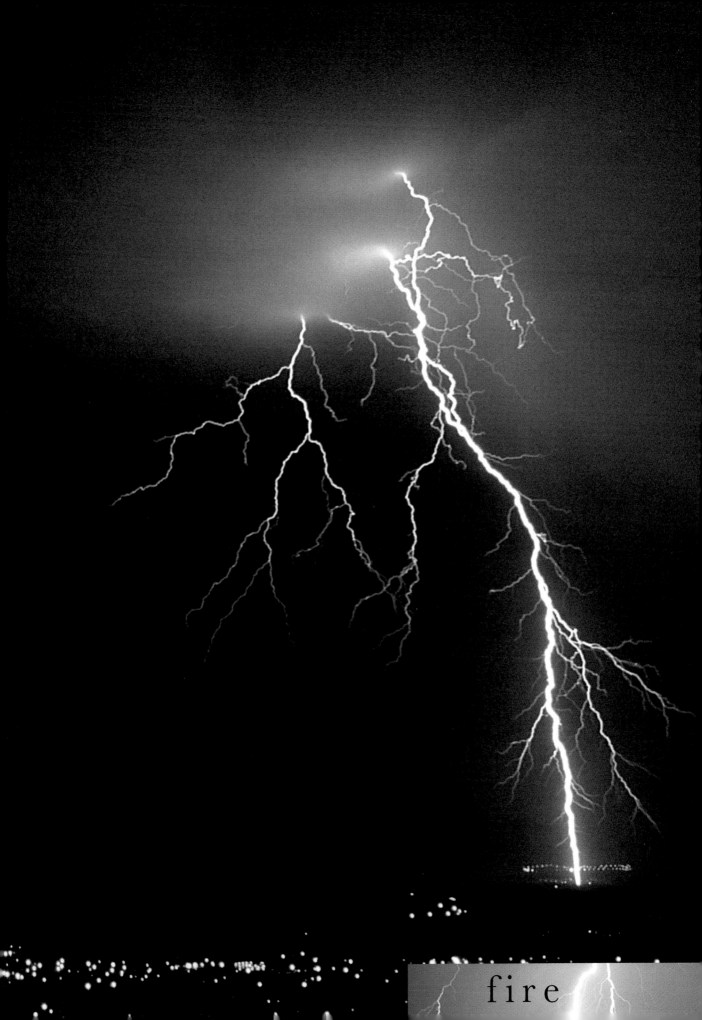

fire

the life force

How often do you have sufficient energy and optimism to relish the challenges that life presents? If you can't remember, perhaps it is time to look at ways of controlling energy-sapping stress.

vital balance

Oriental medicine may have the answer because it emphasizes a holistic or "whole body" approach to health that involves a constant awareness of the body and its needs. Traditional Chinese medicine, for example, believes that the opposing forces of yin (night) and yang (day) create chi (energy), which runs through a system of energy channels, or meridians. Imbalances can be treated by more yin—rest and cooling foods—or yang—activity and heat. In Indian medicine, or Ayurveda, the life force is known as prana. It is taken in through breath and food (which is why Ayurvedic practice emphasizes the benefits of both diet and purging) and accumulates at seven energy centers or chakras, governing the senses, organs, and emotions. These run from the base of the spine to the top of the head (the crown chakra) and need to be kept open and balanced with each other to free the flow of energy and achieve a feeling of harmony.

Indian and Chinese systems of medicine are based on the idea that universal energy flows through the body. In Chinese medicine, the energy follows lines called meridians—acupressure and acupuncture points lie on the meridians—while in Indian medicine energy accumulates at one of seven centers called chakras. Both systems stress the importance of balancing the flow of energy.

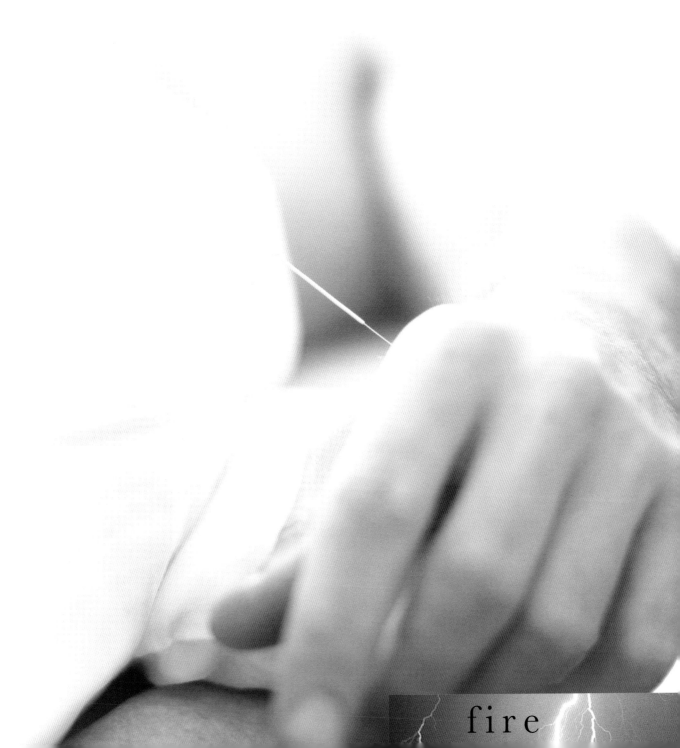

fire

removing energy blocks

An important way to release this vital energy is by touch.
Shiatsu and tui-na, like acupressure (acupuncture without
needles) work on specific points to free the blockages that
can cause ill health. Reiki, on the other hand, is a form of
healing that aims to divert the life force to areas in the body
where its power is most required.

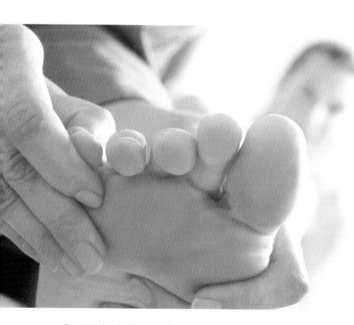

By manipulating various pressure points around the body,
proponents of Eastern medicine suggest they can rebalance
the flow of energy and so treat common problems such as
headaches and anxiety. Two popular therapies, acupuncture
and acupressure, are based on this system.

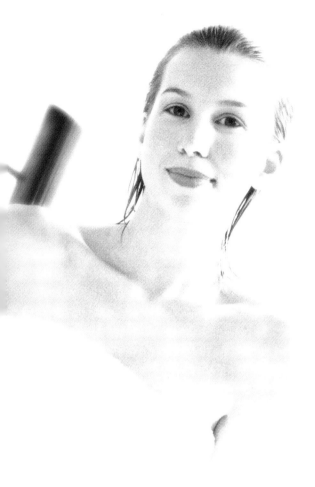

heal yourself

You can use the acupressure points to unwind when you're feeling stressed. To relieve tension headache and anxiety, first press the center of your forehead between the brows with your index finger, then press the base of the skull and the back of the neck. Now push the ball of your foot into the ground. The center of this area is called the Bubbling Spring and pressing it disperses excess chi or activity. Finally, press the top of the foot where the bones of the first and second toes join to revive yourself.

fire

air

From the first gasp to the last breath, air

is the most vital element of all.

Everything we do—the way we feel, think,

and move—relies on the atmosphere that

envelops our planet. The marvellous

balance of gases, which includes the

oxygen necessary to sustain humans

and animals and the carbon dioxide that

allows plants to flourish, is what

makes life possible.

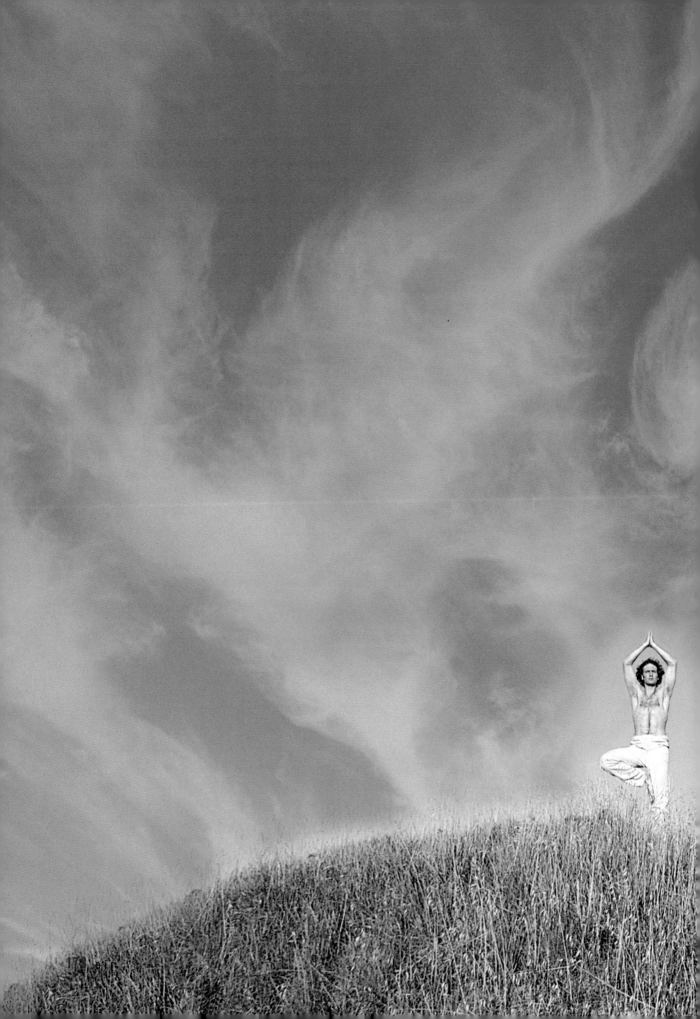

spiritual

Where is heaven? In legend, **paradise** exists above the blue arch of the sky. Although we know that outside the earth's atmosphere lie black holes, cold planets, and burning stars, we still look into the skies and beyond our world for a place of **peace** and contentment.

air

the breath of life

Breath is the source of life and of inspiration (the word means literally to "draw breath"). The moment you take your first independent breath and utter your first cry, your character begins to emerge. Breath not only makes speech and communication possible but also drives the heart, pumping oxygen-rich blood to all of the body's cells, including those in the brain. The way we breathe is fundamentally linked to our physical and mental well-being.

uniting mind and body

Deep breathing is essential for relaxation but it also has a spiritual element. The aim of meditation and yoga is to release the soul, uniting the physical being and higher consciousness by breath control, or pranayama. In Indian Ayurvedic practice, there are five types of prana, (life force) which are linked by a series of energy channels, or nadis, connecting the purest form of prana, which rises from the crown of the head, to the lowest center in the abdomen, which moves down toward the earth.

air

sun and moon breathing

Yogic alternate nostril breathing involves both hemispheres of the brain to balance mind and body, inducing a feeling of deep peace.

Sit cross-legged or in an upright chair, keeping your back straight and eyes closed. Press the thumb of your right hand against your right nostril and breathe in deeply to a count of four. This is moon breathing, which uses the left nostril to calm the spirit.

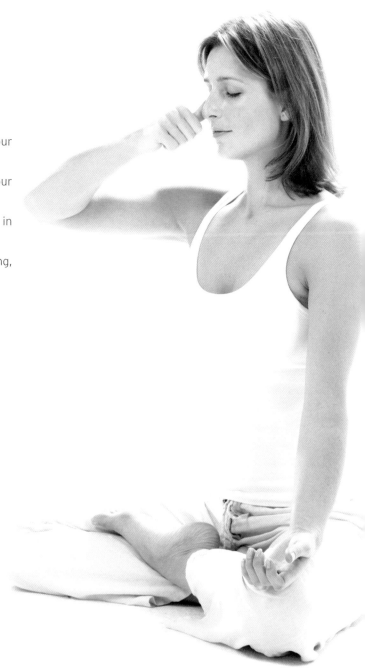

Now alternate it with sun breathing through the right nostril, to increase stamina and energy levels. After taking air in through the left nostril, hold your breath, then close your left nostril with your longest finger and breathe out through your right nostril to a count of eight. Be aware of any difficulties in your breathing. Now breathe in through your right nostril to a count of four, then close it, and breathe out through your left for a count of eight. Repeat three times, increasing daily until you can do seven.

air

the gift of healing

Healing is an ancient tradition. In many religions, a priest's blessing and laying on of hands are thought to convey both physical as well as spiritual comfort. But it is also true to say that many types of healing—psychic surgery, miracle cures, and shamanism—have brought complementary medicine into disrepute.

beyond explanation

What is fascinating is that healing seems to work—not always, not predictably, but often enough to make it worth considering. Skeptics say this may be due to the placebo response—the mind-over-matter effect well known in hospital trials, where dummy pills have been demonstrated to have at least a 30 percent success rate. But research shows that there may be more to healing than this alone.

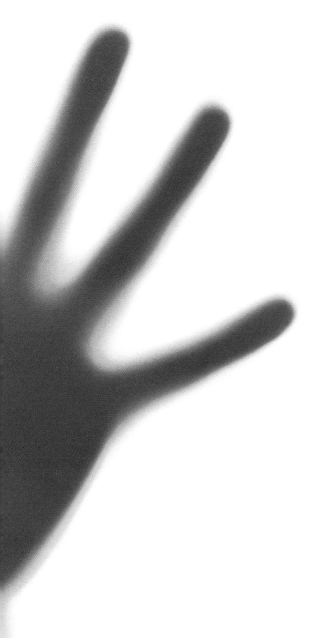

the healing message

Most healers are modest about their powers, saying

that they simply encourage self-healing in sufferers.

Many find that their hands feel hot when they heal and

it is known that their brainwaves can slip into the

relaxed alpha state observed in sleep and meditation.

Both the bodily heat and mindset of the healer can

influence the person being healed, boosting the spirits

and encouraging relaxation. As stress and anxiety are

known to raise blood pressure and damage the

immune system, the comfort that healing can give, by

touch and even prayer, make it an effective way to

rally the forces needed to fight disease.

air

hypnotherapy

You feel relaxed, very relaxed. So much so, that you are virtually unconscious, though you can move when you are directed. In fact, you are in a trance where your personality is totally subjugated to the will of another.

Hypnotism of this kind was made popular by Franz Mesmer in the eighteenth century, and has been followed by thousands of stage acts ever since. But this should not be confused with hypnotherapy. Like hypnotism, hypnotherapy works on the subconscious, but it is more like a peaceful form of psychotherapy. Certainly you should feel relaxed, but you may not even be aware of entering a state of altered consciousness during a session.

implanting ideas

Hypnotherapy is a good way to treat all kinds of addictions, from smoking to negative behavior. It works in two ways, by relieving anxiety and implanting positive ideas that cut through the negative messages your mind may be creating: "I must have a cigarette," "They're staring at me," or "I've got to get out now." This makes hypnotherapy effective for panic attacks and stress-related complaints like irritable bowel syndrome, asthma, and also for pain relief in dentistry and childbirth, by encouraging the brain to produce endorphins, the happiness chemicals.

altering your consciousness

Since you need to have absolute faith in the hypnotherapist, it is essential to choose a recognized practitioner. After an initial visit to a hypnotherapist, there is a lot you can do at home on your own, if you have sufficient insight into your behavior. Spend at least fifteen minutes a day on self-hypnosis if you want to see results. Try the following exercise. Sit or lie down in a quiet, private place; close your eyes and breathe deeply and slowly. Visualize yourself walking along a long path or corridor toward a point of light at the end. Repeat positive statements ("I feel completely at ease," "I love the taste of food now I don't smoke") or listen to them on an audiotape. Visualize yourself turning round and walking back until you reach the room where you are resting. Become aware of your body, open your eyes, and sit up slowly.

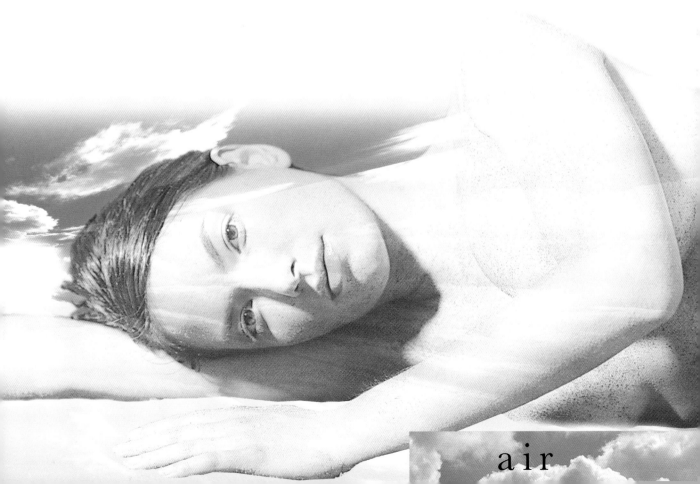

air

think yourself well

Remember the best holiday you have ever had. You were relaxed and at one with the world, right? You loved the country, your partner, and the people you met. Above all, you felt really well. Now ask yourself: Did you feel well because you were happy, or were you happy because you felt well? It is one of the most fascinating conundrums in modern medicine, and prompts the question: If stress makes you sick, can positive thinking make you better?

medicine of the mind

Mind-body medicine is the popular name for psychoneuroimmunology (PNI). PNI assumes that because there is a direct connection between the central nervous and immune systems, thoughts can have a direct, physical impact on the body. Though this approach may be new to conventional medicine, it is the philosophy behind holistic therapies from Ayurveda to zero balancing, which recognize that the brain does not work in isolation. For example, positive thinking is known to relieve pain and can even mimic the effect of drugs. Experiments with chemicals that cause a skin reaction show that a conditioned response occurs even when water is used, pointing to a mental connection.

positive and negative

Stress and depression, on the other hand, release large amounts of a hormone called cortisol into the bloodstream, which weakens the immune system. The right therapy can lower the level, which is why it is vital for cancer patients who suffer from depression, as many women with breast cancer do, to have special help. A "whole body" treatment, consisting of the best that surgery, drugs, psychiatry, and complementary therapies have to offer, is necessary to combat serious illness like this. Our health needs more than a purely clinical approach because we also need to feel stronger and happier in order to be ready to fight illness.

air

positive action

Positive thinking is a start but positive expression is essential too. As with meditation, it is not enough to read about it and understand it. You have to do it. Try...

...other awareness

Connecting with other people is important for maintaining your mental health. Directing your attention outward rather than inward is a key component of confidence and well-being. But why not take it a step further and actively improve life for others? You do not have to be intrusive or interfering—a smile or a greeting can be as effective as flowers.

...self expression

Chanting, singing, acting, gardening, and writing down your thoughts are all ways to create positive emotions. It is more than just the pleasure of accomplishment: In expressing yourself and by creating something, you access your subconscious, which helps you to formulate ideas and articulate half-hidden emotions, fears, and hopes.

...decisiveness

Do it, delegate it, or drop it—this popular business mantra is worth applying to your personal life, because it stops the gnawing anxiety caused by problems that build up and won't go away. If you are constantly tense and on edge, it is worth taking time to work out what is troubling you, with the help of a therapist if necessary. Then either resolve the situation, share it, or accept it, making a list of pros and cons if necessary to help you decide. Role-playing—acting out a scenario with a partner— can be helpful if your courage fails you. But do not procrastinate. It wastes time and saps energy.

...movement

Exercise can improve mood faster than chemical antidepressants and boosts energy levels too. Granted, you do not always feel like exerting yourself, but the endorphin surge really does exist, and you get a toned body too. What more can you ask?

air

stay in touch with your family

Isolation does not come naturally to humans. Everything we do shows that we are naturally social animals, predisposed to live in communities and to interact with each other. Of course, as the French philosopher Jean-Paul Sartre famously remarked, "Hell is other people;" as every city commuter knows, it is easy to have too much human contact. But although people can be a source of stress, research increasingly shows that relationships are invaluable for health and happiness.

family ties

The best gift any parent can give their child is unconditional love. Nothing contributes more to confidence in adult life than the knowledge that you are loved for what you are, not what you can do or what you represent. But families do not always have a benign influence, and missing out on love as a child can mean you have to struggle for self-acceptance later. One way to achieve this is to think back to an incident that upset you. Imagine yourself at the age when it occurred and interview the child you were. Ask yourself what happened and why it mattered. What were your feelings and how did it affect your development? What can you do about it now? Laying old ghosts to rest is a good way to free yourself from bitterness.

air

pet power

Animals can provide solace if you are cut off from human contact. Caring for a pet involves responsibilities and rewards that improve mental as well as physical health, and despite the risk of allergy and infection, studies show that pet owners are generally healthier and live longer than non-pet owners. Some of the benefits are obvious: Walking a dog or riding a horse entail exercise in the fresh air and brings you into contact with people as well as animals. (Oddly, people are far more likely to stop and talk if you are taking a dog for a walk than if you are on your own.) Others are less expected: The rhythmic action of stroking a pet to the sound of snuffles or purrs can lower your blood pressure and probably your pet's too, it also reduces stress after a busy day.

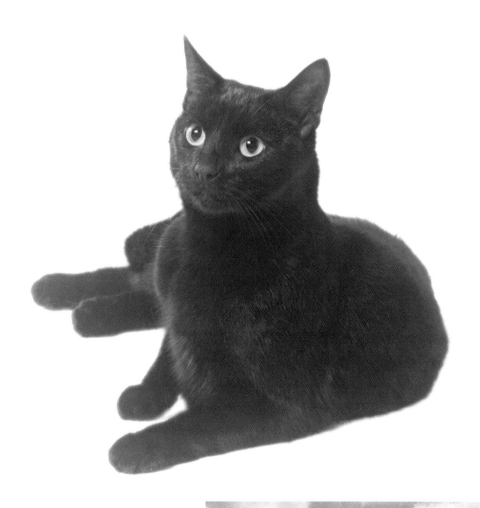

air

widen your circle of friends

Good friends are a joy to be around. They share your interests, help out when needed and provide a buffer against life's mishaps and miseries. No wonder forging relationships is important for mental health.

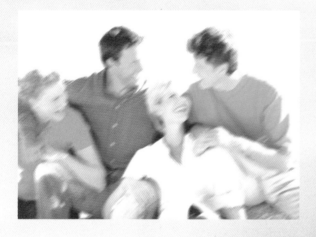

Making friends is an art that can be learned if it doesn't come naturally. Two important factors are to be open minded and to let your defenses down.

social skills

Making friends is an art, but it is one that can be learned. Positive body language and eye contact are two components, and if you are stuck for small talk, try the compliment/question technique: "What a lovely place! How did you find it?" Combine open-ended questions like this, which keep conversation flowing, with a summary of what you've been told to show interest. "You spent three years in Paris... lucky you! What was that like? What did you do next?" And remember to listen to the answers.

personal space

Everyone needs some time on their own—even away from their partner—so solitude can be a luxury. Away from the crowd, you can make time for quiet and constructive thinking, reviewing your problems, refreshing your mind, and getting some perspective.

soul mates

If finding like-minded people is a problem, ask yourself, "What do people like me do?," then follow through. That could take you to a reading group, to amateur theatricals, or mountain walking. Go to singles' meetings and, if the thought appalls you, remember that you don't have to commit yourself, and if you find just one person who strikes a spark, it is worth the effort. And there are other benefits: According to psychiatrists, an open mind and the ability to get on with a range of people are good for mental resilience.

air

touched by angels

Religious belief is good for your health, according to studies in pain at Duke University. And although you might expect religious faith to improve your mental health, what is surprising is that religion can actually improve your physical well-being, too. The question is, why?

Religion can offer hope, a sense of purpose, and a strong network of social support, so you are better able to cope with setbacks. Religious beliefs create optimism, which in turn boosts the immune system. And if you do become ill, your faith could make it a more positive and more manageable experience.

It is important to find a spiritual dimension to life, whether it is via one of the major world religions (Judaism, Buddhism, Hinduism, Sikhism, Islam, Christianity), or through some personal spiritual beliefs. And if you are in need of a guide, who better than your guardian angel?

angel therapy

Angels are messengers that move between heaven and earth. In Catholic

tradition, everyone has a guardian angel and there are said to be 72, roughly

one for every five days of the year. The purpose of angel therapy is to put

you in touch with a spiritual guardian who will bring enlightenment and

assist you with your prayers. To enlist his or her aid, simply sit in a quiet

place and call on your angel for help. Either call them by name (you can

identify your angel via one of the many angel websites) or by function,

calling for the angel of healing or forgiveness. According to angel therapists,

your guardian angel is always close by. Whether you are aware of your angel

or not depends on whether your mind is open to the spiritual presence.

air

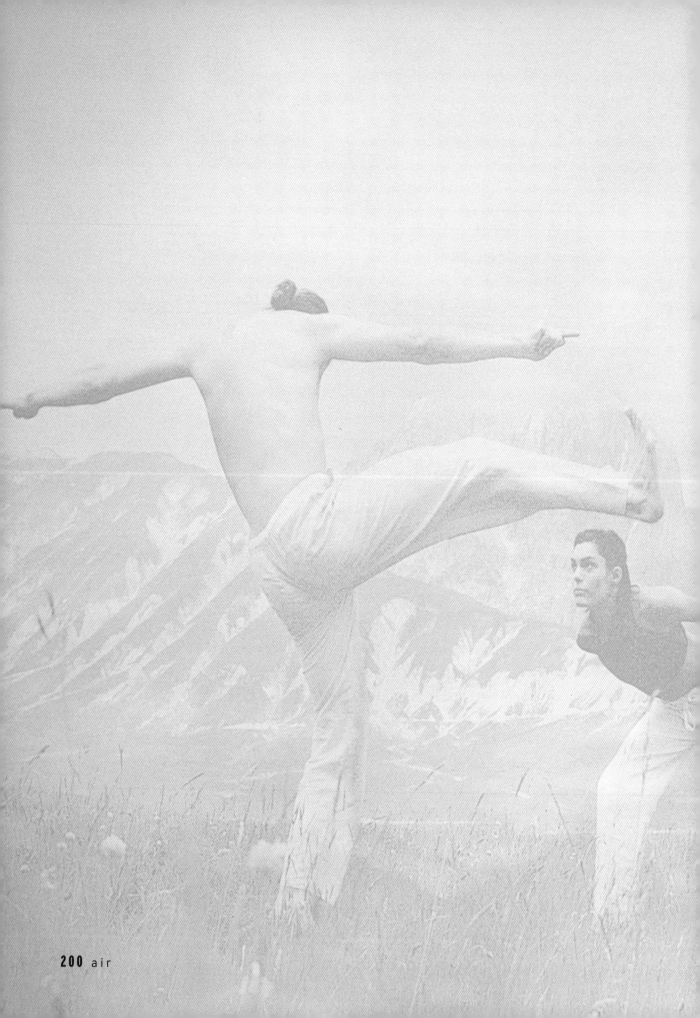

whole

Fitness is more than just physical. Mind, body, and spirit form a trinity, each part of which is an essential element of good **health** and if one is disrupted, it affects the whole. **Restoring** the harmony between them is the key to natural well-being.

air

the art of breathing

Are you an upper-body breather? Breathing quickly so that the chest rises and falls with each breath uses only a

fraction of the lungs' capacity and restricts the flow of oxygen to the vital organs, including the brain. Controlled,

deep breathing slows the pulse and encourages relaxation while also promoting clear thinking.

unlacing the corset

Breathing should inflate the abdomen before it expands the chest. If you find this exercise difficult, lie down on your back and raise your knees, keeping your feet flat on the floor.

Put your hands on your belly and touch the roof of your mouth just behind your teeth with your tongue.

Breathe deeply through your nose, where the cilia—hundreds of tiny hairs—trap and filter impurities. Feel the air flowing through your lungs and down through your body. Expel the air slowly, taking twice as long as when breathing in, then inhale through the nose again so you do not gulp air.

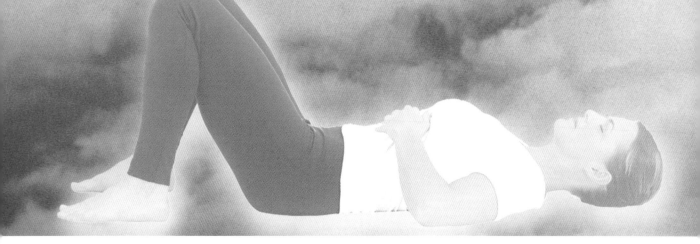

slow the pace

As your breathing becomes slower, deeper, and more controlled, you will begin to relax and feel more peaceful and less stressed. This Zen exercise reflects the natural pattern of breathing, and anything that interferes with it—anxiety, tight jeans, a corset, and bad posture—should be avoided.

Fast breathing can lead to the hyperventilation associated with panic attacks. Breathing into a paper bag to increase exposure to calming carbon dioxide is one way to correct it. Another is by practising the Buteyko method, helpful for people with asthma. To try it, breathe in through the nose as normal and practice holding your breath for increasing periods until you can stop breathing for the recommended one-minute pause. Follow with at least three minutes of normal breathing, but do not try this if you have high blood pressure or heart disease and do not push yourself—the aim is to hold your breath without discomfort or gasping for air.

air

pure oxygen

Oxygen is a natural healer. A powerful disinfectant, it can kill bacteria, which is why hyperbaric oxygen therapy, where high-pressure oxygen is pumped into a sealed chamber, is used to heal deep wounds. And it works: By increasing oxygen supply to the tissues, stimulating disease-fighting white blood cells, and encouraging new blood vessels to form, oxygen therapy can improve wound healing by 70 percent.

fresh air therapy

What is true of oxygen could also apply to its chemical cousin ozone. You can experience this therapy in ozone steam baths and in oxygen bars, designed to counter the effects of pollution, where you can sip an oxygenated drink in the oxygen-rich air to restore energy and clear thinking. Oxygen is in short supply today, especially in cities where levels have fallen from 21 percent to 18 percent or less. We need five pints every minute when we are resting and more than 17 pints when we are active, so we need to top up our supplies constantly, the thinking goes.

wake up your brain

The brain is greedy for oxygen, consuming 20 percent of the body's intake, which is why breathing correctly can sharpen the mind. So too can ginkgo biloba. The leaves of the Chinese ginkgo tree improve circulation by dilating the blood vessels, allowing more oxygen to reach the brain. There is evidence to show that 120 milligrams a day can boost short-term memory, concentration, and alertness, Ginko can cause side effects when taken with other drugs, so consult your doctor first.

air

stillness

A quiet mind, free from anxiety and unhappiness, is the modern nirvana. When was the last time you were really at peace, away from the noise and rush of the crowd and untroubled by agitated thoughts? By rediscovering the lost art of stillness, you can experience this sense of calm whenever you choose. And it only takes 20 minutes a day.

the relaxation response

During meditation, alpha waves flow through the brain, creating a state of mind that differs from sleep and from consciousness. The body is fully relaxed but, paradoxically, the mind becomes more alert. Breathing slows, blood pressure and levels of stress hormones fall, and tension ebbs away. As a result, meditation is frequently recommended as therapy for heart disease, chronic pain, addictions, and stress reduction.

mind clearing

Regular meditation refreshes the mind so you are better able to deal with problems. Freeing your thoughts from

day-to-day concerns gives your mind the space to focus on what really matters. It also encourages acceptance and

an unprejudiced approach to new ideas. When we can look at a situation calmly and without our usual instinctive

emotional responses taking over, we can combine intuition and logic to make good, healthy decisions.

Critics question whether this state of passive awareness can make you vulnerable to manipulation by groups or

cults. It is true that some forms of meditation look to a yogi, or master, like the Maharishi Mahesh Yogi who

developed Transcendental Meditation. But meditation can easily be practiced at home, without a teacher's guidance.

The most important thing is to make time aside every day to do it.

air

3 approaches to meditation:

simple Zen meditation

Many novices find it difficult to sit still. However much you try to ignore your body, it is surprising how quickly you can develop a painful crick in your neck or an unbearable itch. However, there is no need to adopt the lotus position—you can sit anywhere you like that is warm and quiet, though not so comfortable that you fall asleep. An upright chair is fine as long as you feel at ease and your feet are flat on the floor. If you prefer to sit on the floor, tuck a small cushion under your backside to tip yourself forward slightly and make it easier to support your back.

Put your hands in your lap and straighten your back and neck, holding your head as though it is being pulled up from the crown by a string. Drop your shoulders and close your eyes.

Breathe in deeply through your nose, so that your belly swells, then breathe out, feeling the tension drain from your muscles. Repeat several times.

Breathe slowly and rhythmically, counting every time you exhale until you reach five, then start again.

It is worth realizing that sometimes the urge to fidget is an escape mechanism for your thoughts, which tend to wander at first. The trick is to gently bring them back from the world outside. One of the easiest ways to do this is by concentrating on your breathing, a basic Zen practice. By counting every out-breath, you can quieten the intrusive voices that threaten to disrupt your meditation. Focusing on breathing is often the first form of meditation that people try. The goal is gently to empty your head of distracting thoughts and to adopt a receptive silence.

Stop when you are ready—it will probably be after about ten minutes the first few times you meditate. Breathe quietly for a minute before opening your eyes, and then sit still for a further minute.

Stand up and stretch to restore blood flow. You should feel energized and mentally refreshed.

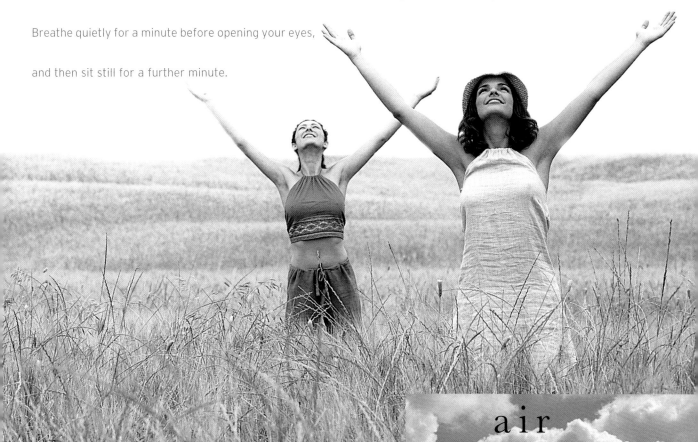

air

3 approaches to meditation:

mantra meditation

There are other ways to concentrate besides counting. If you are a visual person with a tendency to daydream every time you close your eyes, it may help to focus on an object—such as a flower, a handkerchief, or a candle flame—as you meditate. On the other hand, if you find yourself distracted by external sounds or internal chatter, the answer could be to try mantra (chanting) meditation. Energetic people who find it hard to curb their movements can combine mantra chanting with counting rosary beads or spinning a prayer wheel to help channel their thoughts. A mantra can be a word, a name, or a statement of belief. Short, rhythmic phrases are ideal, whether they are Ave

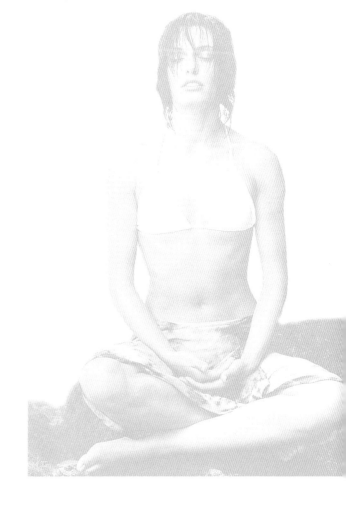

Sit down, close your eyes, and breathe deeply, as with the basic meditation. When your breathing becomes stable, speak the mantra and repeat it, lowering your voice each time until you are barely whispering.

Maria or jiv jago ("wake up sleeping souls"). Some practitioners believe that since the aim of a mantra is to blot out mental static, meaningless phrases are best, while others argue that a mantra should be a short prayer.

The most sacred Vedic word is Om, or Aum, which can be expanded into Om tat sat ("Absolute eternal truth"), but there are many others to choose from. Hare Krishna, Krishna Krishna, Hare Hare, Hare Rama ("O Lord, the supreme truth, I want to serve you") is another well-known Indian mantra. The responses given in the Christian church ("Lord have mercy upon us") can also be used because meditation is part of the Christian tradition, too.

Continue chanting the mantra silently. The sound will seem to vary—sometimes it will seem louder, sometimes further away. If thoughts intervene, brush them aside and return to the mantra.

To finish, breathe deeply several times, moving your fingers and toes. Open your eyes and then stretch.

air

3 approaches to meditation:

mindfulness meditation

Vipassana, or mindfulness, aims for inner peace by different means. Instead of ignoring sensations, it advocates becoming absorbed in them. Losing yourself in the moment—a process called "flow"—helps you let go of anxiety and stills your racing thoughts.

Although mindfulness can be practiced when you are seated, you can use it throughout the day. Instead of fretting over what you have to do as you walk along, slow your pace and become aware of the effect of the sun, rain, or wind on your face and body. Appreciate the movement of your limbs, feel the ground beneath your feet, and listen to your breathing. Do not try to hold on to these sensations; just let them pass and focus on the next.

mindful of the day

Jon Kabat-Zinn of the University of Massachussetts developed a complete stress reduction program based on the regular practice of mindfulness meditation. These suggestions are adapted from his plan to achieve a more fulfilled working day.

Talk to your partner and family before you leave for work—take an interest in their plans and activities.

Be aware of your body and your surroundings as you travel to work and sit in silence for a few minutes before entering your workplace.

Think about how you relate to colleagues and what you can do to improve communication.

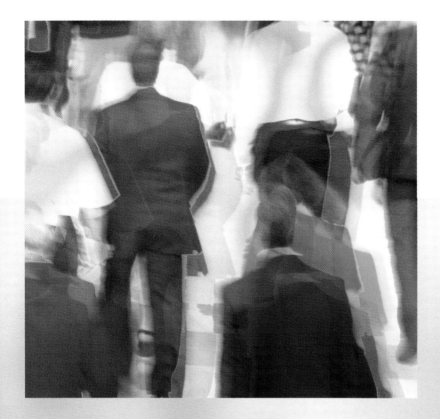

meditation can be used as a
practical tool throughout the day

If you are interrupted when you are working, take a little time to refocus before returning to what you were doing, and don't just rush back into it.

Two or three times a week, unwind by taking a walk during your lunch hour, observing and focusing on the sensations of your body as you move.

Clear your mind and sign off for the working day by making a "to do" list for the following day.

Mentally let go of work during your journey home so you feel refreshed when you return.

Greet your family individually when you arrive home.

Relax—mark the change from one sphere of your life to another by changing your clothes.

air

flexible mind, flexible body

There is bound to be a form of yoga that is right for you. There is hatha yoga, whose reviving stretches are found in every fitness class. To burn fat, try the more active ashtanga, or power yoga, which involves vigorously leaping from one posture to the next, or for spiritual growth try kundalini, which awakens a serpent coiled at the base of your spine, changing awareness as it moves upward.

Yoga activates the chakras (energy centers) along the spine through asanas (postures) and pranayama (breathing control). Yoga means "union" and it is the ultimate mind-body therapy, improving circulation, breathing (even if you have asthma), flexibility, and mood. After a class you should feel happy, centered, and in touch with every part of your body, without feeling tired or breathless. Begin with simple yoga stretches, holding each one for fifteen seconds for maximum effect. Until you are more practiced, avoid advanced postures and mentally challenging forms of meditation. Yoga is a complete philosophy, not just a

keep-fit program, and one that takes time to learn. To

benefit fully from it, you should be aware of the

mental, physical, and spiritual aspects of each asana.

air

release the stress

relax with a twist

This exercise rotates the lower spine and gently works the abdominal muscles. Lie on your back with your arms outstretched and raised to shoulder height, so your body makes the shape of the letter T. Bend your legs, keeping your feet flat on the floor and pressing ankles and knees together. Breathe in. Breathe out and gently lower the knees to one side, keeping your legs together and making sure both shoulders stay on the floor. Control the movement with your tummy muscles and do not force your knees down. Hold the

strengthen your spine

Designed to open the heart chakra, this pose expands the chest and works the upper back. Lying face down, tuck your hands beside your shoulders and place your forehead on the floor. Your legs and ankles should be pressed together. Breathe in, raising your head and look up, bringing your shoulders and chest off the floor. Take your weight on your hands, keeping your head and back straight, but your belly on the floor. Hold for a few breaths. If you feel confident in the pose, extend your arms so your belly comes off the floor. As you breathe out, lower yourself slowly to the floor and rest for a moment. Repeat three times. Relax by sitting on your heels, knees tucked underneath, then stretch your arms forward, touching your forehead to the ground.

pose, then breathe in and raise your knees back to the

center. Breathe out and in.

Repeat on the other side

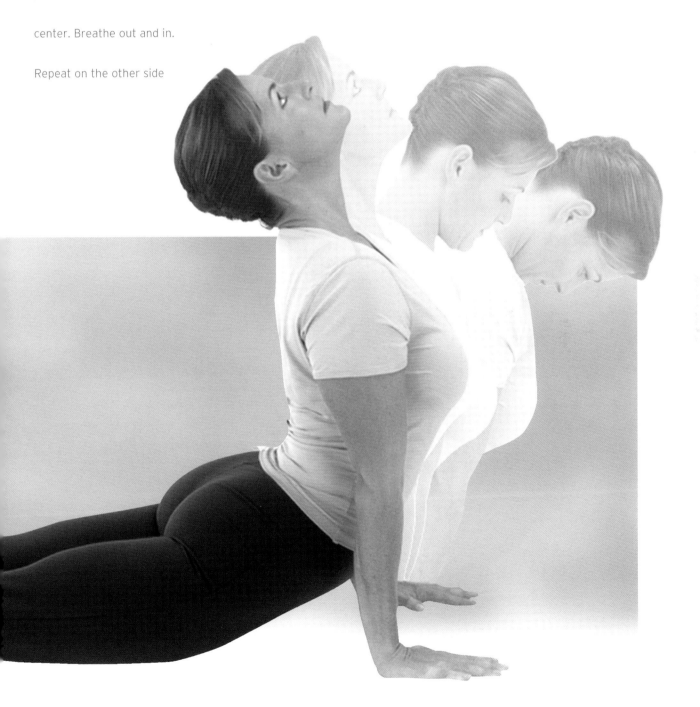

air

the moving image

Where India has yoga, China has qi-gong. Like yoga, it combines movement, thought and breathing to improve the flow of chi—vital energy or life force. The postures of qi-gong and t'ai chi, its dynamic derivative, sometimes called meditation in motion, were designed to be practiced standing, ideally out-of-doors. The moves flow smoothly and are not complex at all. Both are wonderful ways to achieve calm and fend off the harmful effects of stress.

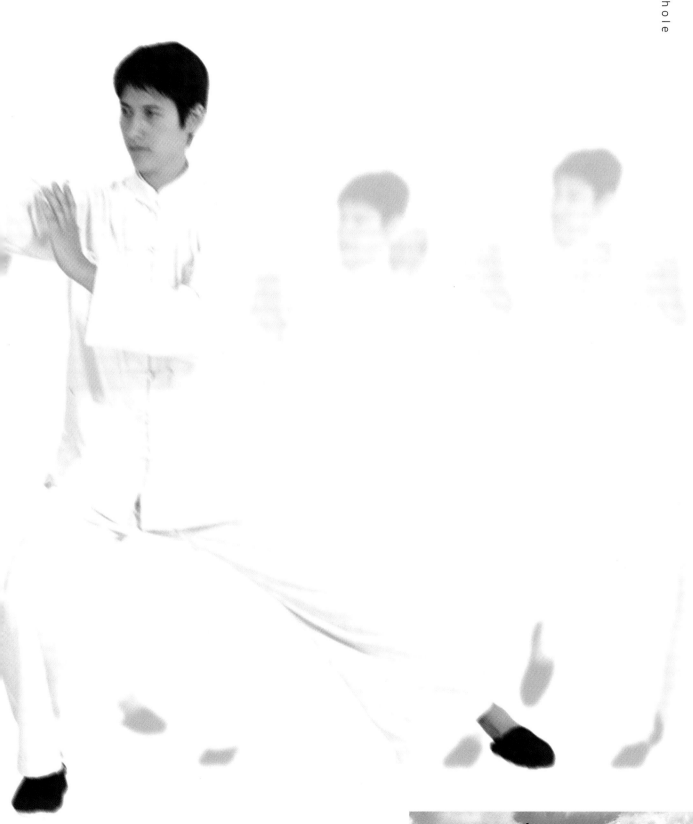

air

cloud hands and drawing the bow

cloud hands

The following simple circular movements will help you concentrate and work the upper spine. Stand in the basic qi-gong position, feet parallel and hip-width apart, back straight, knees slightly bent. Swing your arms and shake your shoulders briefly to loosen up.

With your weight on your right leg, move your left palm to face away from your collarbone and your right palm beneath it, facing up, level with your navel. Twist your upper body to the left, turning your palms so they face each other in the process.

Swap the position of your hands as you move back to the center so that your right palm is level with your collarbone and your left palm is level with your navel.

Return your weight to the right leg, with palms facing each other. Return to the start position.

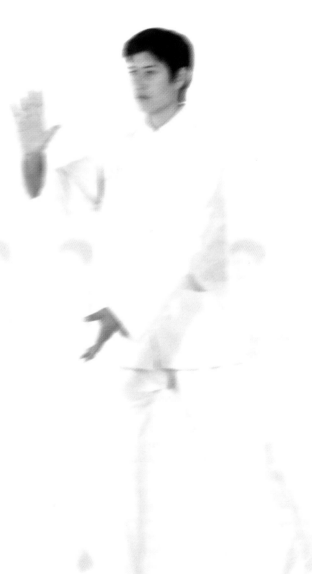

drawing the bow

This easy exercise opens the lungs and gently stretches and flexes the spine.

Stand with feet wide apart, knees bent. Turn your head and upper body to the left, drawing an imaginary bow as you move so that your left arm is extended and the right is bent, level with your chest.

With your left palm facing away from you, flex your fingers and look at them.

Hold the pose for a moment before returning to the center. Repeat on the other side.

air

healing sounds

Translate the frequencies at which the planets vibrate into notes and you will hear the music of the spheres. This eerie symphony is the song of the planets, which shares the same resonance with many sacred sounds, slowing the brainwaves in the same way as meditation to create a feeling of calm.

sound	pronunciation	organ
Xu	shhh	liver
Ho	huh	heart
Fu	who	spleen
Chu	chewee	kidneys
Xi	ssea	lungs

voicing emotion

The six healing sounds of Chinese Taoist tradition connect with the organs of the body and

rebalance the emotions. Some practitioners may interpret them differently but the principles

are the same. Chant them slowly, letting the sound vibrate your lips and palate.

negative emotion	positive emotion
anger	kindness
cruelty	love
anxiety	openness
fear	gentleness
grief	courage

The sixth sound, Hey (ay) restores unity by linking with the "triple burner"—the three

areas governing breathing and circulation, digestion, and reproduction and elimination.

air

the universal mantra

"Om" can be used as a chant in its own right as well as an aid to meditation. Start by drawing

an "Oh" sound deep from your larynx and throat into your mouth. Now widen your mouth,

keeping the lips relaxed, to form a higher "Ah" note. Then close your mouth to make the

humming sound, "Mmm." The sounds represent the trinity of body, mind, and spirit, so chant

each syllable slowly, allowing it to resonate before it merges with the next.

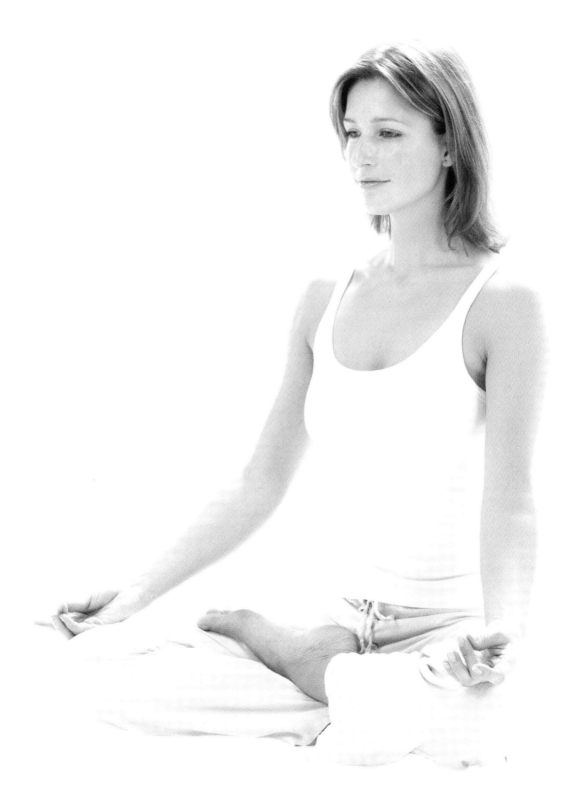

air

balance

Harmony is the secret of good health. Mind, body, and soul are so intimately **connected** that any disturbance in one is bound to affect the others—restoring a healthy **balance** in the way we live, feel, and relate to others is vital for our future happiness.

air

the slow lane

When was the last time you strolled down the street, spent two hours eating lunch or lingered in a garden at dusk, drinking in the scents and sounds as darkness fell? If it sounds like a scene from an old movie, perhaps you need a change. Time stress (which the Japanese call "hurry sickness") sees many of us attempting to do too much, finishing very little, and satisfied with virtually nothing. It triggers the familiar litany of stress-related complaints—such as eczema, migraine, irritable bowel syndrome, and chronic fatigue—which cloud our enjoyment of life, and can depress immunity and trigger heart disease too. So how can you buck the 24-hour, seven-days-a-week society? Time management schemes, with their insistence on accounting for every minute of the day, are rarely the answer. First, see if you can reduce your working day to free up more time. Yes,

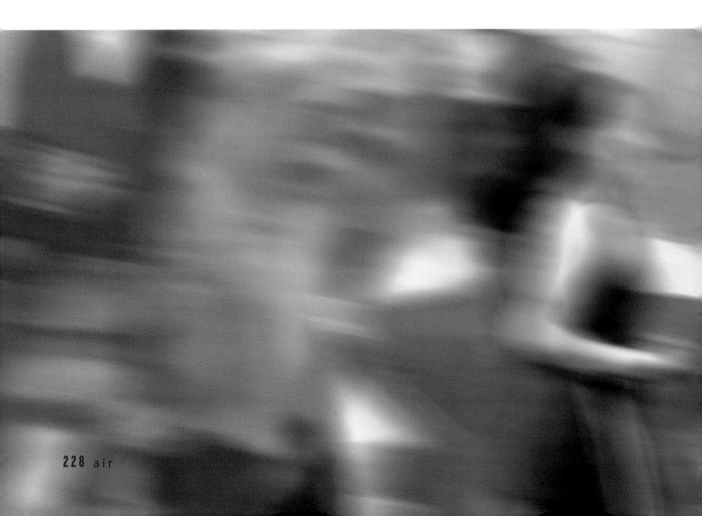

of course you need the money but listen to the British psychologist and work-life expert Cary Cooper. He believes that though working an extra hour a day by choice is not harmful, any more can damage your health. Second, record how you spend every hour for a fortnight. At the end of the time, review it and see if you can spot the energy drainers—things you do that are neither necessary nor enjoyable. Then ditch them.

Third, devote more time and effort to the ones you love. Call up a friend and arrange to go out, take a long walk with your partner, or spend an hour or two putting your children to bed, regularly. Substitute people time for project time and watch your relationships, in all areas of your life, flourish. Fourth, feed your soul. Explore nature, art, music, poetry, or religion—whatever it takes to lift your spirits and lift you above humdrum concerns.

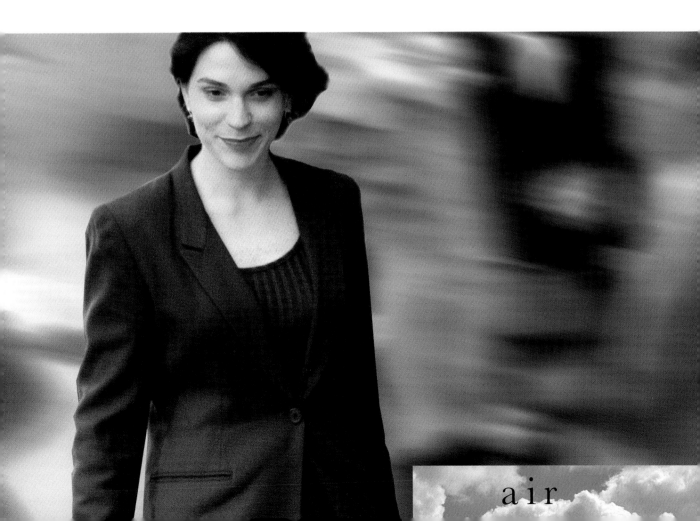

air

enjoy!

Greet the day with new zest by dumping the invisible burden of cares that weigh you down. This is stress, the ultimate imbalance between demands and resources, and its effects are all too obvious.

Stress is cumulative. Being knocked sideways by a stressful life event—dismissal from your job or a relationship crisis, say—dents your ability to cope, and you may find yourself sleeping and eating less, drinking more alcohol and worrying more. As a result, you not only fail to deal with the initial problem but find yourself heading for a major crisis. Chronic stress can impair the body's immune system, triggering panic attacks or stress-related illnesses, or plunging you into depression. But there is a way out. The answer is to reverse the negative spiral by boosting your defenses.

Your body often gives the first signals that you are suffering from stress. If you have a series of colds or unexplained headaches, regularly wake up in the small hours, or lose interest in sex, think about what has been happening over the past few months—writing it down may help. Eventually you may decide to make major changes to your life, but meanwhile there is a lot you can do to increase your resistance to stress.

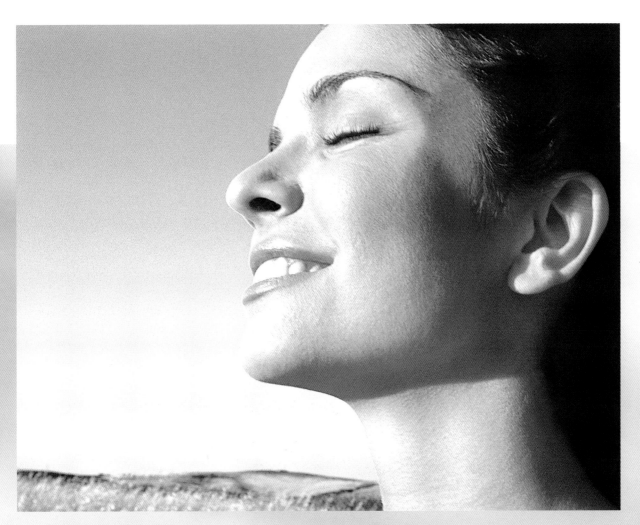

air

helpful thinking

Psychologists have identified thirteen pessimistic thoughts that contribute to stress, from negative thinking ("Everything's going wrong") to all-or-nothing behavior or pronouncements ("Unless it's perfect, it's not worth it") and minimizing ("Even my good points are useless"). To counter them, ask yourself the following questions.

How is this thought helping me?

What is really wrong with my situation?

How will it seem in a year's time?

How would my friends see it?

If I have to leave/give up, what will really happen?

the future is yours

Visualization can help if you are anxious about the future. If you are worried about

an interview or challenging social situation, think about it carefully and visualize

yourself successfully overcoming the obstacles. And if it is the present that is a

problem, try putting it in perspective by imagining yourself a month, six months,

one and five years from now, to see how you could improve your life.

air

free your body

Stress tells the body that it needs to be ready to fight or flee. This state of readiness causes muscles to knot when you are under stress, putting pressure on your bones and joints. Letting go of tension can boost your body's resilience. It only takes ten minutes of progressive relaxation to unwind tense muscles yet the results can be impressive, lowering adrenaline, blood pressure, glucose, and cholesterol in the blood and lactic acid in the muscles. Try the following relaxation techniques.

Lie on your back with your feet apart and hands by your sides.

Tense, hold and relax the muscles in your right foot and leg, one by one, starting with the toes and moving up to the thigh; then repeat with your left leg.

Clench and relax each of your buttocks in turn and contract and release your stomach muscles.

Work the muscles in your hands and arms.

Shrug your shoulders, raising them to your ears several times. Work the muscles in your face, then relax.

Roll your head gently to relax your neck. Feel each muscle in your body easing.

air

instant results

If you are aware of stress building up during the day, you need to take immediate action. Try these quick stress-busters:

Forehead—Widen your eyes, then screw them up and hold the pose for five seconds before smoothing your brow. If you frown unconsciously, psychologist David Lewis advises sticking a piece of adhesive tape across your brow to act as a reminder.

Shoulders—Roll your shoulders forward and back, then shrug them toward your ears, repeating three times. Draw them forward across your chest, then back to bring your shoulder blades together.

Back—Repeat each movement three times. Lie down with your knees raised and pull in your navel so your back is flat against the floor—check it with your hand— then release your abdominal muscles. Now squeeze your bottom and raise it, pulling in your abdominals at the same time. Finally, hug your knees to your chest and raise your head, keeping your back on the floor.

air

the mystery of sleep

Sleep is the natural way to replenish your energy reserves, yet many of us has less than six and a half hours per night. It is a common misconception that sleep is a passive state and that you could make far better use of the time.

Far from it. During the different phases of sleep, stress hormones drop, blood pressure and heart rate slow, and growth hormones surge, which is why kids really do need early nights. And though your brainwaves change, your mind remains active during sleep.

sleepless nights

What can you do if you are one of the millions of people who suffer from insomnia? You probably know all about sleep hygiene, but a sleep routine that re-sets your body clock can be even more effective. U.K. Sleep specialist Professor Jim Horne recommends the following strategies.

What happens when we don't sleep? After a few nights without sufficient sleep, changes in the immune system and symptoms associated with premature ageing, like memory loss and problems handling glucose may occur as levels of the stress hormone, cortisol, rise. But the most dramatic effect of sleep loss is on our thought processes. Creativity, critical judgment, and even the ability to speak clearly and express yourself are affected, and Australian research has shown that lack of sleep can impair drivers' reactions even more than alcohol, already mentioned.

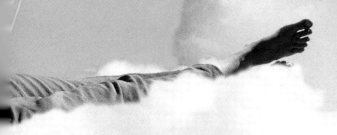

Do not nap during the day, even if you have had a bad night's sleep. Ignore the clock and do not go to bed until you can't stay awake any longer. However late you go to sleep, get up at the same time every morning, even at weekends. If you don't fall asleep within 30 minutes of going to bed (the definition of insomnia) get up and leave the bedroom. Do not read, chat, or watch a late film—all of which are far too stimulating. Opt for a routine activity that occupies your hands and eyes, like tapestry or jigsaws. "If it's 6 A.M. and you're still doing that ridiculous jigsaw, don't worry," says Professor Horne. "You'll be sleepy that day, but stay awake until 10 P.M. and sleep is virtually guaranteed."

air

loving together

Two years is roughly the length of time being "in love" lasts—the feverish state when your whole being is focused on a significant other and you count the moments you're apart. The two-year timespan could well be the reason why there are so many relationships that seem well past their sell-by date. What it does not explain is why we also find couples who have been together for 30 years or more and take as much joy in each other's company as on the first day. One Californian couple I met recently have been together for 53 years. She got married as a nervous 19-year-old but had matured into a feisty, energetic 70-something. He was funny, laid-back, and obviously liked as well as loved her. Everything they did, their body language, the way they deferred to and complimented each other, showed the richness of their relationship.

be good to each other

If you are in a relationship that you want to last, there is a lot you can do to change it from being so-so to so great. Respect is a quality that is often lacking. Are you as careful of your partner's feelings as you are of your friends'? Would you speak to a colleague in the same way? Criticism won't get you far. Remember the child care manuals with their emphasis on positive affirmations—ignore the bad, praise the good. Human beings don't change much and this approach works in adult relationships too.

If you are on the receiving end occasionally, let it go. Tolerance means accepting your partner as a whole person, even the bits you don't much care for, and you should expect the same in return. For why should anyone else value you if you don't value yourself?

Couples who express tenderness verbally as well as physically provide the right climate for love to grow. According to Oxford University happiness guru, Professor Michael Argyle, even using your partner's name can help, because it is a reminder that you have an individuality beyond Mr. and Mrs., mom and dad. But because this is a union too, sharing thoughts, hopes, dreams, activities, and resources is vital. Successful relationships center on good communication, where both partners can express themselves and listen to each other. Above all, have fun and your relationship should be strong enough to cope with the change and challenges you face—together.

air

sexual yoga

Three hours of lovemaking that creates a wave of bliss leading to a whole-body orgasm—not an everyday sexual

experience, perhaps, but certainly one to aspire to. Tantric sex, which unites the teachings of the Kama Sutra with

meditation and bodily control, seeks to extend those fleeting moments of ecstasy when you feel at one with your

lover and the universe. The word "tantra" means to expand, and there are several ways of achieving it.

Best-known, perhaps, is the instruction for men to "cool down" during lovemaking. The idea is to delay ejaculation,

which classic tantra teaching saw as weakening. Frustrating? Not necessarily, because "dry"

orgasms are allowed and exponents report that sexual surfing can be highly pleasurable.

Unsurprisingly, women tend to be wholeheartedly in favor because tantric sex

emphasizes female pleasure and encourages multiple orgasms.

Because sex is seen as the ultimate way of connecting mind,

body, and spirit, ritual is essential. The room should be

prepared with flowers, aromatherapy oils, candles,

and silk drapes or throws. Couples are encouraged to

take their time eating or bathing together, and

Tantric sex encourages couples to focus
on the energy between them and not
just the physical sensations of sex.

give each other slow, languorous massages with essential oils. Only then do they

start to explore every part of each other's bodies in a prolonged foreplay that can

last an hour or more. Because this is a spiritual as well as a physical

union, eye contact is important. But ecstatic "soul gazing"

can also be accomplished by a simple embrace.

air

the tantric kiss

the female partner should take the initiative.

Sit on your partner's lap, with your legs and arms wrapped around him, looking into his eyes. Use pillows for extra support and comfort if necessary.

Start rocking together. Breathe in deeply so that your belly expands, then rock forward, contracting your "love muscle" (your pelvic floor), while he breathes out and rocks back again.

Breathing out, rock back and relax your pelvic floor as he breathes in and moves forward. The rocking motion should become natural and not forced.

Continue rocking as you kiss, merging your breath so you breathe and feel as one. Try to keep eye contact when not kissing, focusing on the feeling of ecstatic union between the two of you.

air

detox your relationships

When a relationship has problems, you have three main options. You can put up with it and wait to see if it mends. You can walk—to the divorce courts, a new lover, or out of your partner's life. Or you can try to heal the breach.

One difficult situation is when a partner or family member continues to behave unreasonably, despite pleas, because the status quo is more attractive to them than the prospect of change. You can see this in addictions like alcoholism, where the whole family may be involved in admonishing the alcoholic, searching for hidden bottles and so on, and this attention, plus the physical dependence on drink, rewards and feeds the antisocial behavior.

In many relationship disputes, a mild form of aversion therapy may work. If, for example, your partner or family won't help with household chores, despite repeated requests, you should simply stop cooking, shopping, or doing the laundry for anyone else but yourself. Be matter-of-fact and do not apologize: "I haven't had time to cook today because I was doing last night's washing up. There's plenty of food in the refrigerator," should get the message over.

It is important to be consistent and to show pleasure when the strategy starts working: "Thanks for putting the dishes

away." Simplistic perhaps, but psychiatrist Raj Persaud goes further and advocates treating people you cannot reason

with as pets. "Reward them when they do what you want and ignore or make a negative consequence when they

behave in a way you find unhelpful," he says.

If you are afraid to take a stand, there may be deeper problems in the relationship, including emotional or even

physical abuse. An imbalance where one partner develops a needy dependency and constantly defers to the other

is unhealthy. Women are particularly susceptible to "learned dependency," where they lose confidence in their

ability to run their own lives. Research shows that self-reliance is an important component of self-esteem and thus

keeps depression at bay, so it is important to stay independent.

air

the laughing cure

You hear a joke, read a one-liner, or catch someone's eye in an overly serious meeting and it starts to bubble up. That's it, you're gone—however much you try to stifle it, what begins as a grin and a giggle develops into paroxysms of laughter that double you up, leave you gasping for breath and make your eyes water. As effective aerobic exercise, laughter is up there with the stair machine and step class.

Laughter has other important health-giving benefits. It decreases levels of stress hormones that interfere with the immune system and increases the activity of natural killer cells vital for fighting disease. The effect can be long-lasting: Recent research in California on volunteers watching a comedy video showed that levels of the antiviral agent gamma interferon stayed significantly raised the next day.

How can you bring more laughter into your life? A sense of the ridiculous is an asset that can be acquired with practice, and it is all the easier in the company of friends. If spontaneous laughter is hard to come by, you could join a Laughter Club and if the thought amuses you, you're already half way there.

Laughter therapy sessions start with deep breathing exercises and yoga stretches and move on to group chants of, "Ho-ho, ha-ha," with hands held high. Guided by a leader, the pace speeds up until the group bursts out laughing. Advanced techniques include hearty laughter, silent laughter, humming laughter (good for the internal organs), greeting laughter, and whole-body dancing or jumping laughter, said to mimic childish glee.

Healing laughter can occur at inappropriate times, because like crying, laughing is a way of dealing with deep and powerful emotion. If your life is bereft of laughter, you may be depressed. Therapy, positive thinking and medication, if you need it, can help bring the health benefits of laughter back into your life.

air

surprised by joy

I once took part in a radio broadcast whose subject was the nature of happiness and whether self-help books could improve your chances of finding it. (The answer from the team of assorted pundits was a cautious yes.) Asked to describe our idea of the perfect moment, most of us were initially flummoxed. One mentioned times spent with family and friends, another art, and I think I volunteered the sense of joy that nature can give, when you see a wonderful sunset, look at the pattern of the waves, or are surprised by countryside unexpectedly laid out before you.

One thing is sure—you cannot manufacture genuine happiness. Indeed, the ability to be happy may be set in our genes, according to a new study at Stanford University, which showed that your general outlook may depend on the way your brain responds to stimuli. While optimists are programmed to respond to images of cute puppies, pessimists, it seems, react more strongly to pictures of guns and spiders.

What you can do is remove some of the obstacles to happiness, which is where this book aims to help. Try this final exercise to open yourself to the possibility of pure, unadulterated, naked joy.

Listen to your body.
Realize that every feeling is preceded by a thought.
Examine these thoughts and decide on their worthiness.

Remember that you are
worthy of being loved.

Find out how to have fun,
because laughter protects
against stress.

Live in the present.

Connect with other people.

Learn to let go.

air

useful addresses

Acupuncture Today
PO Box 4139, Huntington Beach,
CA 92605 4139
Tel: 714 230 3150
Website: www.acupunturetoday.com

American Association of
Professional Hypnotherapists
4149-A El Camino Way, Palo Alto, CA 94306
Tel: 650 323 3224
Website: www.aaph.org

American Botanical Council,
PO Box 201660, Austin, TX 78720
Tel: 512 331 8868
Website: www.herbalgram.org

American Counselling Association
5999 Stevenson Avenue,
Alexandria, VA 22304 3300
Tel: 703 823 9800
Toll-free: 800 347 6647

American Institute of Homeopathy
801 North Fairfax Street, Suite 306,
Alexandria, VA 22314
Tel: 703 426 9501

The American Yoga Association
PO Box 19986, Sarasota, FL 34276
Tel: 941 927 4977
E-mail: info@americanyogaassociation.org
Website: www.americanyogaassociation.org

The American Zen Association
New Orleans Zen Temple
748 Camp Street, New Orleans,
LA 70130 3702
Tel: 504 523 1213
Website: www.gnofn.org

Canadian Sleep Institute
300, 295 Midpark Way SE,
Calgary, Alberta, Canada T2X 2A8
Tel: 403 254 6400
Website: www.csisleep.com

Federation of Natural Medicine
Users of North America
www.fonmuna.org

The Gerson Institute (Holistic Therapy)
1572 Second Avenue,
San Diego, CA92101
Tel: 619 685 5353
Toll-free: 1 888 4 GERSON

Hazelden Renewal Center

(Chemical Dependency and Related Disorders)

15245 Pleasant Valley Road,

Po Box 11, Center City, MN 55012 0011

Tel: 651 213 4000

Toll-free: 800 257 78100

Website: www.hazelden.org

Hypnotherapy Training Institute

4730 Alta Vista Avenue,

Santa Rosa, CA 95404

Tel: 707 579 9023

Toll-free: 800 256 6448

Website: www.hypnoschool.com

International Institute of Reflexology

5650 First Avenue North,

PO Box 12642, St Petersburg, FL 33733 2642

Website: www.reflexology-usa.net

Mental Health Association of Colorado

(offers Seasonal Affective Disorder treatment)

6795 East Tennessee Avenue, Suite 425,

Denver, Colorado 30334

Tel: 303 377 3040

National Institute of Ayurvedic Medicine

584 Milltown Road, Brewster,

New York 10509

Tel: 845 278 8700

Website: www.niam.com

National Qigong Association

PO Box 540, Ely

MN 55731

Tel: 218 365 330

Website: www.nga.org

Stott Conditioning (Pilates-based exercise system)

2200 Yonge Street, 1402 Toronto,

Ontario, Canada M45 2C6

E-mail: stott@stottconditioning.com

Tel: 416 482 4050

Toll-free: 1 800 910 0001

Website: www.stottconditioning.com

The Yoga Alliance

120 South Third Avenue

West Reading, PA 19611

Tel: 010 376 4421

Toll-free: 1 877 YOGAALL

E-mail: info@yogaalliance.org

Website: www.yogaalliance.org

index

acknowledgments

The publishers would like to
thank the following for their help
with the photography for this
book:

The Elliott Brown Model Agency,
Bili Keogh,
Scully Whittington-Brown.

The publishers would like to
stress that information given in
this book is not a substitute for
medical advice. The elderly,
pregnant and those with a
medical complaint should consult
their local medical practitioner.